ON THE OTHER SIDE OF FEAR

VISITS WITH THE SNAKE,
CYBORG IMPLANTS & GREEN PEES.

MY THOUSAND-DAY PROSTATE CANCER STORY

Cliff Whitney

Copyright © 2022 Cliff Whitney
All rights reserved.
ISBN: 9798843274757

CONTENTS

ADVANCE 5
RECOGNITIONS 8

CHAPTER 1.   CATS IN THE CRADLE AND GIFTS FROM YOUR FAMILY 11
CHAPTER 2.   WHAT IS THIS PROSTATE THING? 13
CHAPTER 3.   YOU CAN'T WAIT TILL IT ISN'T HARD ANYMORE TO BE HAPPY 16
CHAPTER 4.   PSA, A NEW KIND OF PUBLIC SERVICE ANNOUNCEMENT 19
CHAPTER 5.   THE FAMILY CURSE 21
CHAPTER 6.   THE C-WORD AND YOUR RISK NUMBERS 23
CHAPTER 7.   BATHROOM WALLS AND A SLAP IN THE FACE 25
CHAPTER 8.   VIAGRA COMMERCIALS AND VISITING THE SNAKE 27
CHAPTER 9.   TV IN THE BATHROOM AND A MOTORCYCLE TRIP 31
CHAPTER 10. MY MOST TRUSTED SOURCE FINDS DR. SCOTT 36
CHAPTER 11. A TRIP INSIDE THE FISH TANK 38
CHAPTER 12. PROSTATE SIZES AND PIRADS LESIONS 40
CHAPTER 13. DEBRIEF AND THE CANCER CONVERSATION 42
CHAPTER 14. I DIDN'T KNOW WE WERE KEEPING SCORE 45
CHAPTER 15. OPTIONS AND CRITICAL DECISIONS 47
CHAPTER 16. THE DAY OF CUTTING APPREHENSIVE BUT CONFIDENT 50
CHAPTER 17. THE THING MEN FEAR THE MOST 54
CHAPTER 18. TIME FOR A BEER BUT WTF IS THIS? 56
CHAPTER 19. BLADDER CONTROL AND KEGELS 58
CHAPTER 20. GRADUATIONS AND A TRIP TO CELEBRATE 60
CHAPTER 21. MORE CANCER, MY BROTHER DIES 63
CHAPTER 22. BABY DIAPERS AND CARRYING A LOAD 66
CHAPTER 23. GETTING THE GUN OUT, I SIMPLY CANNOT GO ON LIKE THIS 68
CHAPTER 24. TEN PADS A DAY & MEETING DR. AVALON 70

CHAPTER 25.	MOTORCYCLE TOURING AND PEEING ON BUSHES	72
CHAPTER 26.	LOSING A CHILD AND MAKING DECISIONS	75
CHAPTER 27.	NO OTHER OPTIONS SO SUCK IT UP!	78
CHAPTER 28.	CAMERAS UP YOUR PENIS	80
CHAPTER 29.	INSTALL DAY, I WOULD APPRECIATE WAKING UP	82
CHAPTER 30.	I'M ONE OF 5000 OUT OF THREE MILLION	84
CHAPTER 31.	GREEN PEAS AND UNDERSTATEMENTS	86
CHAPTER 32.	ACTIVATION DAY, I'M NOW A CYBORG	89
CHAPTER 33.	WHAT I FOUND ON THE OTHER SIDE OF FEAR	91
ABOUT THE AUTHOR		94
ENDNOTES		96

ADVANCE

I'm not a doctor, nor do I even play one on TV. I am a total stranger to you, and we will most likely never meet in person. But over the past three years, I have garnered quite an experience with the ramifications of men's prostate health, specifically mine, including battling the dreaded "C" word.

I don't care what kind of person you are: executive, man on the street, macho, timid, in great shape, obese, great attitude, or a total ass. When you are told you have cancer, when you hear those words for the first time, it will mess with your head. This is life-changing news and even the most fearless of us will shake at hearing the word. Cancer is associated with the destruction of lives, pain, and, sometimes, means death. In your mind, during the dark times, which you could have, and which for me I kept to myself, my self-talk was what my younger brother Scott always told me, "This too shall pass."

The text on the following pages is for informational purposes only. Any medical terms, facts, figures, and opinions (which I have a lot of) that are listed here are mine. In no way, shape, or form should anyone use this short read as medical advice, diagnosis, or treatment of cancer. My intent in sharing this story is to archive my thoughts and remembrances on my experience, partly for my own mental health, but more so to share my story with those who could be enduring prostate cancer or those who want to grow their education (especially men).

Further to this, my hope is if you are contemplating action for your condition, especially surgery to remove your prostate, you will learn and get educated, really educated, on your options. I share here my story, what happened to me, before, during, and now after multiple surgeries, and an AUS implant that you will learn about later in this text. You should fully understand what the ramifications "could" be if you decide to go forward.

This text is embarrassing, very explicit, and an extremely personal subject. It is hard to talk about, much less write about or publish, but share I will, a little about myself, my family, and my journey's timeline. Now that my ordeal is over (I hope), I will also give some perspective as to what I might have done differently or should have learned more about before decisions were made.

Doctors, nurses, and surgeons are indeed miracle workers. I have such great admiration for these folks who have the skill and confidence to cut someone open, hold an internal body part in their hand, and repair, replace, or remove it. I have even more admiration for those who do it correctly!

Just think about that for a minute; imagine performing ultra-delicate surgeries on another person. These are extraordinary folks who will have a special place in heaven. Be aware, however, that these folks with ultra-cool technical skills and calm hands don't necessarily translate to the best communicators nor are their answers always right. Even if they are right, things can go wrong, and, in my case, did. Thankfully I was blessed to have had the best of the best when it came to doctors and nurses. I remind you however that Doctors are practicing, and it says so right on the sign, the Dr. XXX's medical practice. We mere mortals need to translate surgical talk into a language we can all fully comprehend and then make our own decisions based on all the information we can gather. Those decisions can be tough, and stressful, and even when making all the right decisions, things can still go wrong.

If you learn anything from my experiences, my hope is you will use it to spread the word to bring more awareness about this type of cancer and then make your own decisions that will better your health.

Again, I am just a guy, a total stranger, so hopefully I can tell a story that is worth telling and encourages you, and others, to do your research, get tested often, and make good decisions so you can keep living LARGE!

As I left my surgeon's office after the activation, I walked down the long hallway with the fancy hospital carpet and out into the parking deck. About halfway down the long line of parked cars, I clicked the key fob and opened the door of my 2008 Toyota Tundra. It was a stretch to get up and in, and even at 6 ft 2 inch., I grabbed the handle just inside the door, which was up high on the left side of the driver's compartment. From there, I pulled myself up and stepped into the cab. It was a long high step, and I paused as I sat down in the seat. I had lost count of how many times I had been poked and prodded. I have had so many things cut on and shoved up every orifice of my body, but for the first time in almost 1,000 days, and under the strain of pulling up to get in my truck, I was amazed I did not pee in my pants.

RECOGNITIONS

I am sorry my sweet wife had to travel down this road with me, but I am blessed you did. I love you so much and am thankful you suggested my second surgeon. In our 40+ years together, you have always been right. Your ability to approach life's challenges with a caring and positive outlook inspires me. I have no doubt that God put you in the right place to make the suggestions that have changed our lives many times now. Without your direction to stop my procrastination and you making me go see the surgeon, the five to seven years of good life expectancy he spoke of would be past the midpoint now. There is a lot I still want to see and do, and while there are ramifications and now some limitations to my abilities due to what I have done to myself, decisions were decided, and the light in your eyes made the ordeal more bearable.

My first doctor almost killed me. So, I say to him, you picked this profession, so get some bedside manner and speak with better words to your patients. Encourage them to get into a good mental state. Have patients repeat things back to you. Disclose everything, in detail, before the fact. Offer up better data, in writing, and take the time to educate your patients so they will make the needed time to read and study the medical information. Then you should spend more time with these folks; don't be in such a rush. Folks like me are coming to you for guidance because we do not know what we are facing and are most likely scared. We need some compassion and all the data so we can make better decisions. You failed at this so do better.

To my prostate surgeon (whom I will call Dr. Scott), I am so happy we got together. You have saved many lives, including mine. You, sir, are a blessing, and there is a special place in heaven saved for you. You, are the best of the best. You took the time, were not in a rush, answered my questions, and then told me the answers to questions I had not asked. On top of all that, I was never pushed, and your processes and methods were on track. Every decision made and the diagnostic results given were pointing me toward the path I ended up deciding to take. I am blessed that your hands, those controlling that monster of a robot, were steady during my procedure. Good karma and more importantly, God, will always be with you.

To my AUS surgeon (whom I will call Dr. Avalon), it is so hard for a man to come to a female doctor and pour their mind out with private issues. Yes, it is indeed embarrassing, but you made it comfortable. I was most likely your worst patient as by the time we met, I was doing a lot of studies. The AUS surgery worried me much more than the removal surgery. After we first met, it took me a year to decide to move forward, but you were there, meeting with me multiple times, virtually and in person, all during COVID and while pregnant too. You answered all my questions, even after I had been on the forums and thought I was an expert. I will not lie; the recovery from your surgery was tough, but the result is a blessing and has given me my life back. During our first meeting, I told you I did not want to cough while you were holding my privates in your hand, but you insisted, I coughed and yes, I peed on you, and yes, I was embarrassed beyond all I know, but you didn't even blink or say a word, most likely until I left the office. ;-)

Thanks so much to the most excellent patient access specialist at the hospital and doctors' offices. You are the first contact, the front line, and I know you never get any credit, but you are special because surgical patients see you first. Your smiles and kindness set the tone for us on very scary days, and we notice. Nursing staff IMO are the same as doctors. You are, however, the ones we rely on once the cutting is over. God bless you.

To my anesthesiologist, your schooling is hard and impressive. I don't know how you did all that school time and are still so young. I always woke up from my surgeries, and I thank you for that.

To the associates at my business, you folks are the best of the best. Each of you knows that the hardest thing for me is to miss work. You did not bat an eye and kept the place thriving while I was out multiple times to heal. When I have the privilege to speak to a group of young people, the advice I give is to surround themselves with successful people and with you folks at the shop, I know I have done just that.

Thank you Blair Townley, we have never met in person nor even spoke on the phone and I am so thankful for the unbelievable job you did line editing my scribblings. I have zero experience in writing so I put the 20,000 words on paper, tried to tell a good story and then read it and corrected it a thousand times over several months, still I knew I needed help (lots of it). While searching for that help I'm sure it was God who guided me to you. I reached out blindly, and to be honest was kind of scared to push that send button as it is hard to take that step and show your words to a real author and editor. You were so kind, offering encouragement in addition to providing fantastic ideas on the arrangement and I thank you.

CHAPTER 1

CATS IN THE CRADLE AND GIFTS FROM YOUR FAMILY

The 1974 song "Cats In The Cradle" is a folk-rock song by Harry Chapin from the album *Verities & Balderdash©*. It is a song I love and sing to when I am in the truck (by myself). It's a sad song, but educational, as it has many lessons about family and the lives we live. It is also about the things we inherit from our mothers and fathers. In my case, I inherited a little high blood pressure and the family curse.

It is now 2022 and in just a few months, I turn sixty-three, am recovering from having prostate cancer, and recently had an artificial urinary sphincter (AUS) installed in my body. Growing up, it was never even remotely in my imagination that I would or could get cancer. Neither was it my intent to be turned into a cyborg, but here I am.

The fact that I am typing this is a good thing. I am blessed not to be one of the 34,000 men who will die this year; however, I procrastinated for far too long, and it was close.

Prostate cancer is like a long emergency. The cancer could take a long time to even alert you that it is present, and you may never even know you have it. The other can just pop up and kill you quickly.

After traversing this health issue, this nightmare, or maybe I should call it a blessing in disguise, I have started thinking about the path I took, the research I did, and the many decisions I made along the way to better understand this enemy. I was constantly asking myself if I was making the right choices. Was I given all of the right and necessary information by my doctors? Was there anything being held back, to maybe make me feel better? Did I ask all the right questions, at the right times, to enable me to make the big decisions? What had I missed, and now that it is close to being over, I wonder, was there anything I could have done differently, or earlier, for a better outcome?

More so, is there anything I can now do to pay it forward and help others, like tell my story?

I still have thoughts in the back of my head that if I had done nothing, I would be just fine, but I also know that if I could see the future clearly, I would not be writing this.

CHAPTER 2

WHAT IS THIS PROSTATE THING?

There is no known way to prevent prostate cancer. In the United States, data suggest it is the second leading cause of cancer death in men after lung cancer, which my brother Scott died of just a short time ago. Estimates are that over 34,000 men will die from this disease during 2022 in just the United States alone. So if you are diagnosed with prostate cancer late, and it has spread to other parts of your body, the five-year survival rate is 31%. For those of you that are not math-inclined, that is an almost 70% chance of dying. [1]

The prostate is a gland in men that helps make semen, the fluid that contains sperm. The prostate surrounds the urethra, the tube that carries urine out of the body. As men get older, their prostate grows bigger, and resistance is futile in terms of stopping the growth.

An enlarged prostate is also called benign prostatic hyperplasia (BPH). BPH is not cancer but still is a curse as it makes you feel like you must urinate all the time and keeps you in the bathroom and in most cases has a big impact on your everyday life. BPH does not appear to

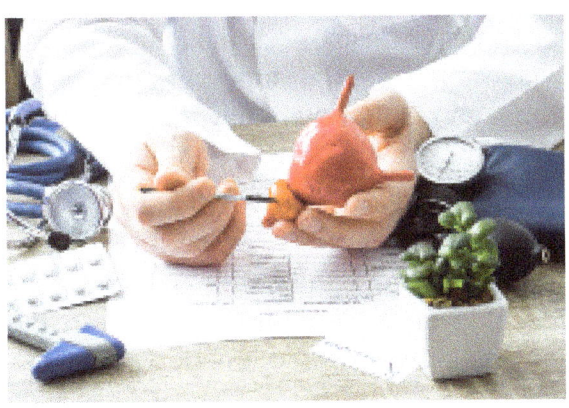

increase men's chance of getting prostate cancer. But the early symptoms are the same as prostate cancer so early testing is critical.

Some of the signs that indicate needing a urologist are:
1. A frequent need to urinate, especially at night.
2. Trouble starting a urine stream or making more than a dribble.
3. A urine stream that is weak, slow, or stops and starts several times.
4. The feeling that you still need to go, even just after going.
5. Small amounts of blood in your urine.

Severe BPH can cause serious problems, urinary tract infections, and bladder or kidney damage.

Cancer, on the other hand, begins in the cells of where your cancer is. Around 400 BC, Hippocrates is said to have named masses of cancerous cells *karkinos*—Greek for "crab." Why a crab? If you feel a malignant tumor, you'll notice that it's hard as a rock. And so, it is thought that it reminded him of a crab's hard shell. [2]

Generally, your body will make new cells when you need them, replacing old cells that die. However, sometimes this process can go astray, and new cells can grow even when your body did not ask for them. On top of that, the old cells may not die when they should have. These extra cells can form a mass called a tumor. Tumors can be benign with no cancer or malignant, where you say, "Houston, we have a problem." If they get aggressive, cells from malignant tumors can jump on and invade nearby tissues in the body. They are nasty, little bastards that can also break away and spread to other parts of our bodies. (This is big trouble.)

Most cancers are named for where they start. For example, lung cancer starts in the lung and breast cancer starts in the breast. The spread of cancer from one part of the body to another is called metastasis (me·tas·ta·sis), which is not a good word to hear.

I never thought I would need to learn so much about cancer nor would I have ever imagined that I would experience it.

CHAPTER 3

YOU CAN'T WAIT TILL IT ISN'T HARD ANYMORE TO BE HAPPY

Once I found out I had cancer I stated feeling somewhat depressed, it was not a good time for me. What helped me get my head right, was when I started being more aware of other folks who were struggling with health issues or who were handicapped in some form and were living their lives to the max despite their conditions. In June of 2021 as I was trying to decide on my next steps, I was browsing the internet one night and heard a young woman, a singing artist who goes by the stage name Nightbirde talking. She said she had breast cancer and had a 2% chance of survival. She was so optimistic and said that "2% was better than 0". This really got my attention, then before she sang, she said, "It's important that everyone knows that I'm so much more than the bad things that happen to me... You can't wait until life isn't hard anymore before you decide to be happy."

When I heard that, I started looking around at things a little differently. I started seeing folks a lot worse off than me with serious issues and they were happy. With this, I was able to talk myself up and away from that place of darkness. I started learning what I was up against and how to finish fixing it.

My first remembrance of the words "PSA test" was from my best friend Anton. We were in our early- to mid-twenties and he told me he was recently at the doctor and had a PSA test done. He said it in one of those passing afternoon conversations where we were out and about and all over the conversational atmosphere, most likely damaging our brains with the heathen devil weed. His comment did not really resonate with me and quickly changed to other more pressing subjects of the day, most likely girls or the size of the universe and wondering if things could indeed be so small that little worlds of people could live under the plants and grass. Hey . . . it was 1979, and the times were the times.

We lived in Charlotte North Carolina, and I was getting ready to graduate out of high school, by the skin of my teeth. My hair was below my shoulders, and I was working three jobs. I was a baker third shift for a donut shop then delivering early morning newspapers and was then driving a school bus in the early mornings and in the late afternoons. In the in between times I was doing my best to go to school and sleep (sometimes in school). My girlfriend at the time, whom I have 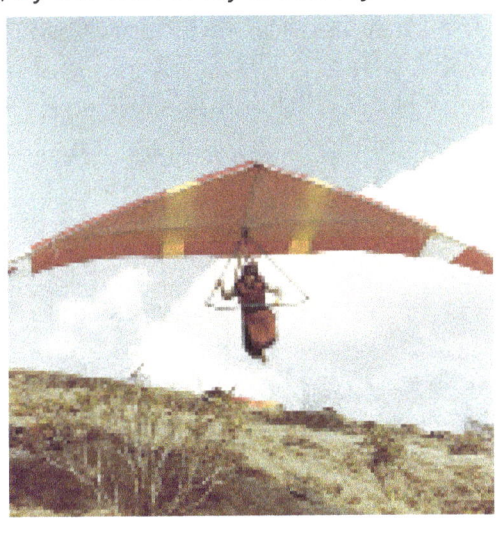 now been married to for forty-one years and whom I think wanted to see more of me in the sunlight due to my nights working, suggested I apply for an advertised job with a young start-up photo equipment retail store called Wolf Camera at SouthPark Mall.

We didn't call them startups back then, but being I was the high school yearbook photographer, and being as I was tired of working the third shift delivering newspapers and baking donuts at the local Granny's donut shop all before driving the morning school bus for the elementary and middle school students, I applied. After somehow passing the polygraph exam, I got the job as a part-time camera salesperson.

As most of us are at that age, I was young and fearless, riding dirt bikes, hang gliding, going skydiving, flying home built experimental motorized hang gliders, hiking and even driving that school bus which always needed some duct tape to keep going. Even today, I encourage my children to explore the world while they are young. After having cancer and multiple surgeries, I see the world in a different light now and push them to travel and experience our world even more.

During this, my high school years and just afterwards, my friends and I traveled to the mountains of Boone, North Carolina each week, where I flew my hang glider off Grandfather Mountain and Tater Hill, with altitude gains of over 12,000 feet. With my new job, I was able to travel many places, including the Hawaiian Islands where I was blessed to fly the hang glider with my young wife tandem off Makapuu Point and then a wonderful flight off the 10,000 ft. Haleakala Volcano that makes up the island of Maui.

Over the next twenty years while at Wolf Camera, the company took on several forms. I worked hard and received many awards as a salesperson and store manager. Then I was promoted to district manager, regional manager, vice president, senior vice president of new technology development, and then, simultaneously, I started and was elected to be the president of the Wolf company Dot com called Wolfexpress, where in addition to selling photo equipment online I was working with a team to develop the technology that allowed photographers to share their photos on a new thing called the internet. With a talented team of associates, we built that small startup into a powerhouse of over 700 stores across the United States.

I had no college education or fancy degree, however the time I spent delivering newspapers and in the photography industry with Wolf and Wolfexpress awarded me what I consider a high-end business degree that you just cannot get in college.

But something I was not aware of was also growing, inside of me.

CHAPTER 4

PSA, A NEW KIND OF PUBLIC SERVICE ANNOUNCEMENT

PSA is a substance made by the prostate, standing for prostate-specific antigen (antigen meaning toxin or other foreign substance). A high PSA level "could" be a sign of prostate cancer, but high PSA levels can also mean noncancerous prostate conditions, such as an infection or BPH. A PSA test is a blood test that measures the level of PSA in your blood.

Most types of prostate cancer grow very slowly. It can take years or even decades before any real symptoms show up. Treatment of slow-growing prostate cancer is often not needed as it grows so slow and might not ever affect you. Many men with the disease live long, healthy lives without ever knowing they had cancer. Treatment, and I can attest to this, can cause major side effects, including erectile dysfunction and urinary incontinence. Fast-growing prostate cancer is less common, but much more serious and, yes, it can kill you.

Your age, family history, and other factors can put you at higher risk (like me), so a PSA test (a simple blood test) is a tool used to screen for prostate cancer. However, there are a lot of reasons some medical groups and even doctors will say PSA tests are not the only option to screen for cancer. My doctors told me that the PSA test by itself can't tell the difference between slow- and fast-growing prostate cancer and this is the reason I did so many other types of tests.

Why get a PSA test?

To find out if a PSA test is right for you, talk to your doctor, but my advice is, if you are over forty, just get tested; after all, you have nothing to lose and a lot to gain. I would get a test once a year during your yearly physical or doctor visit. The reason I suggest routine testing is so you will have a benchmark to judge against. Statistical data is good information, and these statistics will help you make better decisions and stay ahead of the curve if anything does come up.

What happens during the test?

Your doctor will take a blood sample from a vein (easy-breezy), and the test usually takes less than five minutes, with results in a couple of days. Note that you should avoid having sex or masturbating for twenty-four hours before giving the blood, as semen can raise your PSA levels and you don't want to freak out!

When you get the results, a PSA level under 4 ng/ml is generally considered normal, while levels over 4 ng/ml are considered abnormal. High PSA numbers "could" mean cancer or a noncancerous condition, such as a prostate infection, which could be treated with some antibiotics. A high number could also mean nothing.

Age-Adjusted PSA Levels look like:
- 40 to 49 normal is 0 to 2.5
- 50 to 59 normal is 0 to 3.5
- 60 to 69 normal is 0 to 4.5

When I first started having issues and got tested, my PSA never showed results below 4, instead it was climbing.

CHAPTER 5:
THE FAMILY CURSE

The family curse popped up and made me aware of the word prostate when I was in my early thirties. I was living several states away from my folks but heard via Mom that my father, who was in his early fifties, had started having urinary infections. After a couple of years of procrastinating, his urine flow had been reduced to a point where he was up and out of the bed every hour or two, and soon he was having a hard time going at all. My mom mandated he see the doctor or find another bed, so he reluctantly made the dreaded appointment.

Technology being where it was at that time, his doctor recommended a widening of the urethra. Dad told me, "I had to wear a catheter and bag for almost a month before the operation." He also got a shot that he says gave him hot flashes. He spent two days in the hospital, but after a few days of resting up, he said, "Everything was better."

That surgery lasted him nearly fifteen years, then his new urologist noted quite a bit of narrowing again. The doc did an in-office test, inserting a lighted tube for inspection (more about this procedure later). Dad got another "roto-rooter" operation and said, "This time it was easier. I don't remember being catharized before the operation. Only going home the next day with one and removing it in the shower." Dad went back for a post-op check-up about two weeks later and everything was fine, except, on close inspection, a very tiny amount of cancer cells was present. His doctor said it was nothing to worry about, and that the cancer was a very slow-growing type and wouldn't be a problem.

I now wonder how that doctor knew it was slow-growing.

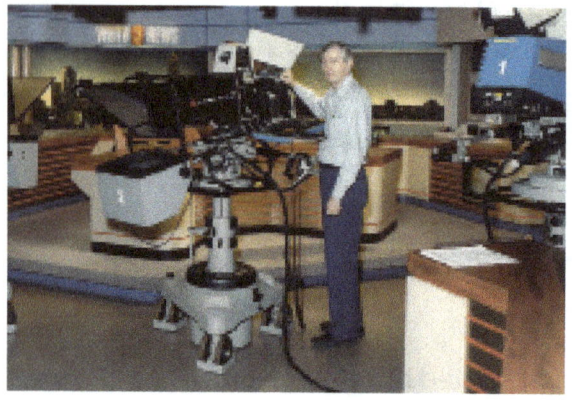

When you are living away from your loved ones, you don't see the daily trials and tribulations of individual family members. Most members of your family, if they are like mine, will downplay their ailments. Knowing what I know now, Dad's surgeries were tough. Surgery is something I don't wish on anyone, especially when you are talking about having a drill bit shoved up your penis.

Dad is now in his upper eighties, and is an artist and video editor for his church. He is still strong and has a very sharp mind, even after quadruple by-pass surgery a few years after his prostate surgeries. He sees his urologist about every six months and recently told me, "Everything is still good except my PSA is up some." He tells me the higher PSA is nothing to worry about at his age and that he is fine.

CHAPTER 6

THE C-WORD AND YOUR RISK NUMBERS

During my visits with my doctors I was told that our risks for prostate cancer include:

1. A father or brother with prostate cancer
2. Being African American. Nobody knows why but prostate cancer is more common in African-American men.
3. Your age. Prostate cancer is more common in men over the age of fifty.

If your PSA levels are higher than normal and you have some testing history in your file, your doctor will more than likely order another type of test, a prostate exam also called the dreaded finger-up-the-ass exam. For this test, your doctor will insert a gloved finger into your rectum to feel your prostate, but this only allows them to feel if your prostate is enlarged. I suggest not making jokes or animal sounds during this test. Remember, this test is indeed embarrassing but more than likely more so for the doctor than it is for you.

Another type of test called a biopsy could also be ordered. Looking back, my experience shows me that this procedure is normally done after you have some history with several PSA tests to establish a baseline or after a prostate MRI. The biopsy is an outpatient surgical procedure, where a doctor will take a small sample of prostate cells for pathology testing. I have had three of these: one very detailed where I was put to sleep and two where I was awake (o' the joy). It is performed with what looks like a flexible aluminum tube being inserted up your ass and the surgical tool has a head that resembles that of a snake. When it opens to take the sample, the tube looks and acts like the monster in the movie *Alien*. Once inside you, the tube opens and a small needle will punch through your colon into your prostate and grab a sample. The doctor will take a bunch of samples all over the prostate or in specific areas where a previous MRI tells them to look.

From talking to my many doctors, the goal of researchers is to develop a test that does a better job of indicating the difference between non-serious, slow-growing prostate cancers and cancers that are fast-growing and life-threatening.

After my experiences with the snake, I am all for that!

CHAPTER 7

BATHROOM WALLS AND A SLAP IN THE FACE

I can't say I was aware I was having issues with my prostate in my late thirties, but now looking back, I remember staring at the bathroom walls a lot more frequently. I didn't think much of it then, and this was most likely due to the partying and a few to many beers with friends, which would keep you in the toilet more frequently.

I was having the time of my life, living LARGE with a hefty salary, a private jet at my disposal, and a wife whose job at Delta airlines allowed us to fly free when we could not get a ride on the company jet.

By the year 2000, I had retired from the photo business and vowed never to work for another person ever again. So, I took the advice from a good friend (thanks Doug) and seeing an industry in change started my own business, an internet only specialized hobby shop out of my home offering electric remote controlled aircraft. I drew on the education from my former photo company life, as I knew how to run a business and, more importantly, I knew how to build an online business and then build a retail presence. I did, and my new shop was growing quickly.

However, in 2006, the term prostate cancer jumped up and slapped me in the face in a personal way. One of the greatest hang glider pilots in the world, and a good friend of mine Rob Kells, announced he had aggressive prostate cancer that had spread. He started speaking on the subject via our national

Hang-Gliding magazine and encouraged everyone to go and have a simple PSA test. I had heard the word PSA before from my friend Anton in high school, but now, and being older, his words gave it some actual meaning.

Unfortunately, my friend's life was cut short—not by a hang-gliding accident, as is often the case, but by cancer. Rob died in August, 2008, and at that time he was only four years older than me.

I was shocked and sad to lose a friend so quickly. Something in the back of my mind was telling me I should be paying closer attention to these new words I was learning. The other side of my head said these things just don't happen to me, and, once again, life was moving fast; time passed and procrastination took hold, again.

CHAPTER 8

VIAGRA COMMERCIALS AND VISITING THE SNAKE

At a normal yearly doctor visit, I mentioned having to go to the bathroom more frequently, and was up a lot, 2-3 times at night. On questioning, I mentioned my dad's issues from years earlier. My doctor prescribed Tamsulosin©, also called Flomax©, did a PSA test, and made a referral to a local urologist in his network. He also told me he wanted to do a prostate exam before I left. This, I learned, was medical code for the ignominious act of shoving a lubricated gloved finger up your ass.

I saw the suggested urologist on August 11 2015. He had two locations and when I got to his business office, we sat down for a chat. He said my PSA test had come back at 5, informing me that was a high number and the only way to see or further test for anything that could be wrong was to do a needle/punch biopsy. Not knowing what this was or what was involved, I said, "You are the doctor. Sure thing, set it up."

As I was getting up to leave, he said he wanted to do a prostate exam. From my previous doctor and the dreaded finger experience, I knew what this was going to be. This is an undignified procedure in multiple ways, and even more so depending on who is administering the poke. My first doctor was respectable and went slow. This fellow was brutal; I could tell by his face, as he squeezed the lube out of the tube onto the paper towel, making sure I saw it. His face started to smile to himself I felt. I think he took great pleasure in this torment and that he enjoyed the anticipation of hearing the gasp as he shoved that finger up someone's ass. However, I did not give him the joy of even a flinch!

What is a biopsy?

A transrectal biopsy is the most common method of performing a prostate biopsy. During the procedure, surgical instruments are inserted through the rectum into the lowest part of the large bowel. Once inside, it involves inserting the biopsy needle through the wall of your rectum to reach your prostate. It will then cut and remove around 10-12 small samples of tissue from the prostate.

I returned a few days later for the biopsy test. This location was different, from his first office. To me, it looked like a Viagra© commercial. In the waiting room, there were posters everywhere, and all the men in the waiting room had their heads down, looking at the floor. Each would head up to the little window when their names were called and leave with a small bag, of what I guessed was Viagra© never raising their heads.

A very nice, attractive young lady escorted me back to the room where the actual procedure would take place, the procedure of which I still really knew not much about (yes, I was dumb and not doing my homework). The hot, little nurse told me to strip and lay on my side on this cold aluminum table, pulling my knees up to my chest. The doctor came in, and I then noticed a rack with what looked like an aluminum hose with a diamond-shaped head about the size of a quarter. As he reached for it the head resembled a rattlesnake. I started to worry!

This guy had the bedside manner of a rock, as he had shown with the finger test. With no real communication, the next thing I knew he had his left elbow pushing downward pressure on my hip and was shoving that thing up my ass with his right hand. It was at that point I was fully introduced to what the words needle/punch meant.

When it was over, he just disappeared, and the young lady said, "You can get dressed and head out." I got up and noticed there was blood all over the table and on the instrument now back in its rack. Looking around, there were no towels, no paper towels, or even a cloth, so I walked out with my cheeks sliding and squishing together with all the lube in that area. I was also sure I was bleeding out the ass. As I walked out, I could see the doctor in his office. With his door open, he looked up, and just as I was going to ask what was next, it appeared he was saying with his eyes, "What the hell do you want?" so I just left.

A week later, I returned to his office a little apprehensive. I almost wanted to run but needed the results. After waiting a long time, he popped in and announced I was good but said, "There could be something there," so he wanted to do the biopsy again in a couple of months. I started to wonder about this guy's motivations and questioning what was up with all this medical technology. These things were not fun, so did this happen to a lot of people with my issue of having to pee often? Nevertheless, on October 20 2015 a couple of months after my first, I went back to the same cold aluminum table and faced the snake, again.

On October 30, ten days later, I went back for the second set of results. The doctor came in, sat down, and, after a long period of his head down, staring at the floor, which I think he was enjoying and which can stress a person who has just a little bit of info, he said, "Well, the good news is you don't have cancer."

To that, and in my best Forrest Gump voice, I replied, "Well, that is one less thing I have to worry about." He replied, "There is something there, but I would not worry about it. It will grow slowly, and you will most likely die of old age before you are affected." After this statement I was kind of shocked that you could have "something" growing inside you and not be given any further treatment, advice or even prescriptions. I reluctantly thanked him for the torture sessions and went on my way, as this guy was no conversationalist.

The two treatments with the snake cost me money out of pocket. I was self-employed, and my insurance deductibles were high to keep the cost down, so I had to pay cash out of pocket, and, as I recall, this fun with the snake and a wacko with slippery hands was $6000 per visit.

I can assure you that playing with the snake is not my kind of fun.

CHAPTER 9

TV IN THE BATHROOM AND A MOTORCYCLE TRIP

Almost a year later on August 13 of 2016, I went to a new female primary doctor and after bloodwork was done, it was learned my PSA was at level 5.

In March of 2017, again at my regular doctor, my PSA was 6. She looked at my chart and ask how it was going with Dr. Torture, 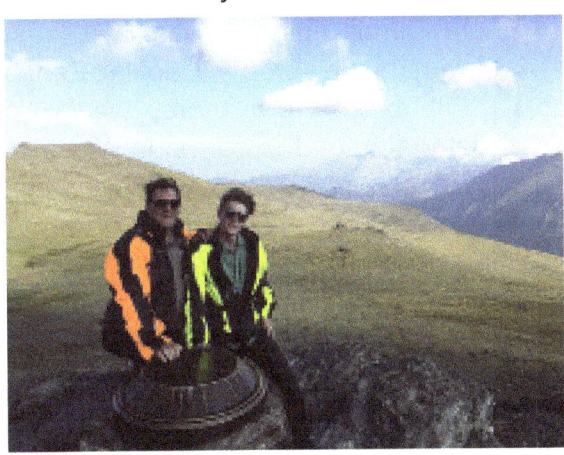 the urologist, as she was looking at the PSA trend on my chart. I told her if I was her, I would never refer patients to him, as he had the bedside manner of a rock. I also mentioned I only thought he was excited about certain portions of his chosen profession, like taking pleasure in torturing his clients. I announced I was not going back to him but I was to the point where I was going to have to install the TV in the bathroom.

On November 7, 2017, my PSA was 8.9. This got my attention, but again I procrastinated and did nothing.

On June 16, 2018, my PSA was 5.3. It was at this point I started to wonder if there was any solid science to these PSA tests.

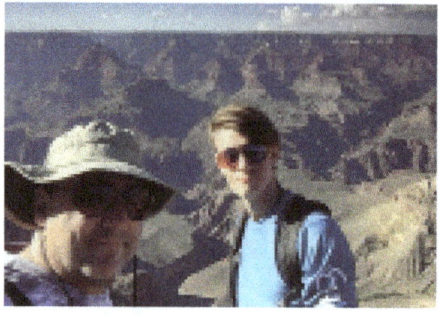

In July of 2018, I took a three-week motorcycle trip as a present to my son Eli, who had just graduated from college early and with honors. We took our brand new 26 ft. class C camper that I had purchased specifically for this trip, along with a custom Ironhorse motorcycle trailer, and hit the road for a month of fun.

I was not in the best of shape, so celebrating was tough. I could not do a lot of walking or exercising due to living in the bathroom every hour or so. But celebrate we must, so off we went.

During the trip, the plan was to stop in a town, camp, and ride the bikes for a couple of days, then move on. After driving south

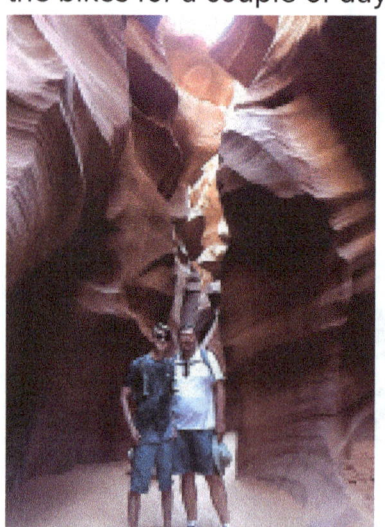

to Birmingham, it was I-40 west with the first stop at Cadillac Ranch in Texas. From there, we were standing on the corner in Winslow, Arizona and out to Meteor Crater. As we were driving along, and with no specific timeline, we took a fork in the road and ended up in the spectacular Monument Valley for a night of camping under the most incredible sky. From there, we cut across the desert seeing no one for hundreds of miles to Lake Powell for a few days at Antelope Canyon, Horseshoe Bend, and a long drive to the Grand Canyon, getting back to camp very late at night. The next day, we were off to Zion National Park, and then another long ride through the desert to Vegas, baby.

TV IN THE BATHROOM AND A MOTORCYCLE TRIP

We road over the 9,043 ft. Tioga Pass to the gates of Yosemite where we were informed the park was closed the day we got there due to the Ferguson wildfire in the Sierra National Forest, Stanislaus National Forest and Yosemite National Park in California so we rode back over the Tioga pass and headed to Lake Tahoe instead. A few days later we then rode over the mountains into San Francisco and across the Golden Gate Bridge.

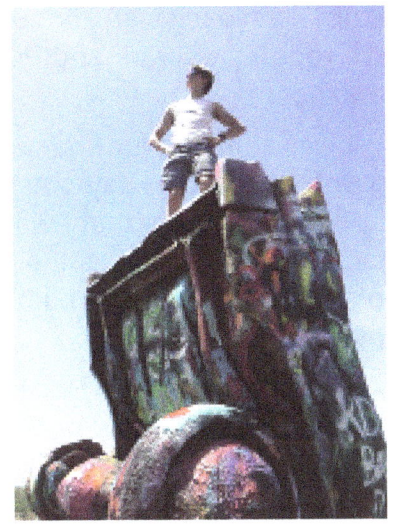

Even though I was having to stop every few hours for nature calls the California coastline north of Mendocino County was so spectacular. The ride had beautiful rocky cliff faces and dark sand beaches. There was lots of fog one morning and on a tip from someone camping next to us the very twisty ride from Willits via 20 over the mountain and through the tall Redwoods was breathtaking, especially following my son, who had no fears riding his graduation present, a new BMW 1200 GS.

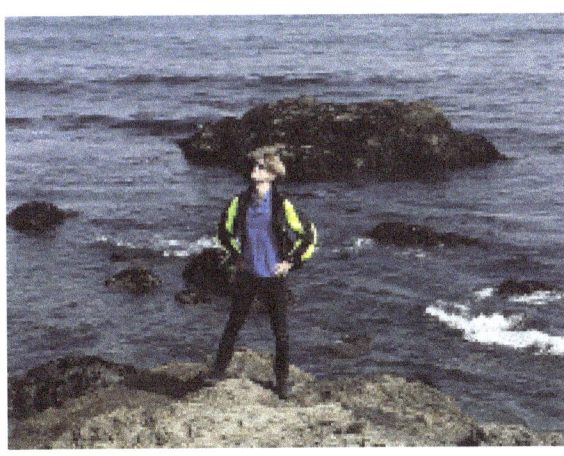

We rode up the coast and then back over the mountain range on an unmarked single-lane road that was even more twisty fun. If you blinked, 200 miles had passed, and that California coastline was so juicy with spectacular views at every turn! We intersected 101 and headed north to Oregon to see more of the big Redwoods, even getting to drive through one of the massive trees. From there, it was on to Grants Pass, where we cut across Oregon, Wyoming, and then Salt Lake City where we had a flat tire in the middle of the interstate at rush hour. We stopped in each state for epic rides and adventures. In Colorado, we rode Estes Park and Pikes Peak before heading back east and home.

It was so much fun sharing these rides with my son, but it was tough and, as they say, cramping my style! It was becoming more and more evident that I was going to have to address the issue of having to visit the bathroom every hour or so.

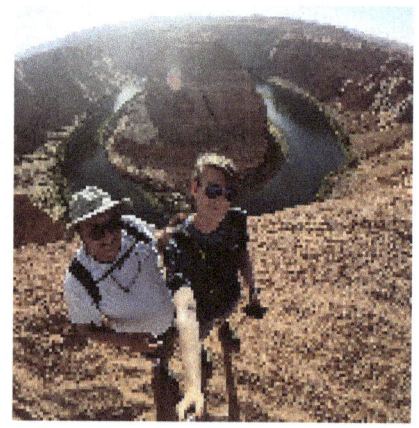

Five months later, on December 7, 2018, my PSA was again 5.3, but it was at that point I was contemplating moving the TV into the bathroom. I was dehydrated due to not drinking enough water. If I drank more that caused the need to go even more often. The Tamsulosin pills were not doing anything for me bathroom-wise, but they were giving me blurred vision and sometimes flu-like feelings as side effects. These effects of the drug had also affected me on our motorcycle trip and blurred vision is no fun on twisty roads. On the upside, my blood pressure was lower due to the drugs.

Being that I thought of myself as an internet genius, I started to study my condition more seriously. Having to be in the bathroom every hour or even more often if I decided to have a small sip of water was affecting my quality of life. I was active as a pilot and on my motorcycles, but long trips were now out of the question or took a lot of planning for bathroom stops. I loved going out with friends; however, everywhere I went (even before I went), the first thing I looked for or gave consideration to was the bathroom.

TV IN THE BATHROOM AND A MOTORCYCLE TRIP

Heck, if I knew where we were going for dinner, I would sometimes look up the restaurant's inside photos on the web to see where the bathroom was to be ready. I was up at least four times a night having to go and not sleeping well.

I was starting to ask myself, *Is everyone my age like this and just not saying anything?*

CHAPTER 10

MY MOST TRUSTED SOURCE FINDS DR. SCOTT

In late 2018, my wife was no longer with the airlines and, after some schooling, was working at a local hospital as a Patient Access Specialist II. As my condition continued to worsen, and after she overheard me mumbling about installing the TV in the bathroom, she told me in early 2019 of a surgeon on her campus that was supposed to be one of, if not the best, urology and prostate doctors in the United States who specialized in robotic surgery. From what she said, and I think she had been doing research, she learned that doctors from all over the United States who had prostate issues came to see this gentleman for help. I learned that he has done more than 250 robotic surgeries a year and had a very long list of surgery first, as well as a page full of awards stretching years.

With this data from my most trusted source, the wife, she made the appointment to be sure I would go, and I first saw Dr. Scott on February 19, 2019. Dr. Scott presented a great persona to me and as I sat in the room with him, I could tell he was a kind man.

During that first office visit, I told myself I liked this guy. He had a great, relaxed conversation with me, and I got the impression that he was a meticulous surgeon. He pulled out prostate models and posters, and I could tell as we talked that he was excited about his work. Never was he in a rush at all to move to his next appointment, and he was confident but not cocky. Looking back

MY MOST TRUSTED SOURCE FINDS DR. SCOTT

and now, knowing this man better, he has every right to be very cocky but instead is as humble a man as I have ever known.

We talked about my issue, my businesses, and hobbies, and his hobbies too, which overlapped somewhat with mine as we were both into drones. All the time during our meetings together, I knew he was busy and in very high demand, and that his time each day was parsed out to get the most done, but this man took his time with me. He was just a nice guy and suggested the next step was to gather a quick PSA test but more than likely, knowing my history and previous PSA results, he said he would need more data; that involved a trip to their new MRI machine. He said that it worked well seeing the prostate in detail and from all angles.

He did a PSA test, and the results were back at 1:09 pm the next day. They showed my PSA was 9.3, with the standard range being 0-4.

Something was indeed growing inside of me.

CHAPTER 11
A TRIP INSIDE THE FISH TANK

On March 19, 2019, I went for a visit with the tube, aka the MRI machine. Before I went to have the test done, and due to my previous visits with the snake, I had done my homework researching what an MRI was on the internet and knew what was going to happen.

The facility was simply beautiful, with furnishings nicer than my home. I was escorted back, and the young nurse apologized jokingly for the office not having designer robes, as she handed me a skimpy thing of a robe. Once dressed, she took me into the room where the massive machine lived. You could hear the monster humming with the anticipation of looking inside me.

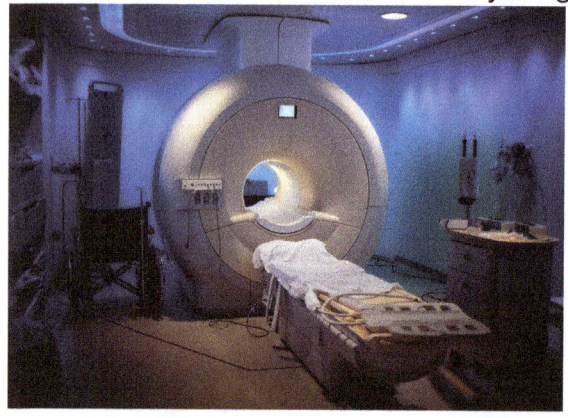

The operator, a nice, young lady, walked me over to a control panel and suggested I pick out some atmosphere and music. *Music?* I thought. "This is no spa," I said as a joke. She stopped me and said, "Watch this." She punched up some soft soothing music and the entire room transformed into what I can only describe as a fish aquarium, and we were on the inside of that aquarium looking out. The walls were covered in many kinds of

A TRIP INSIDE THE FISH TANK

tropical fish that were swimming all over the walls and ceiling, as the lighting transformed the room into soft blues and greens. This was so cool, so I climbed in, put in my earplugs and headphones on, and received a device on my head to look at, this showed me the fish while I was in the tube. It was so restful I took a nap in the aquarium while the machine pounded away.

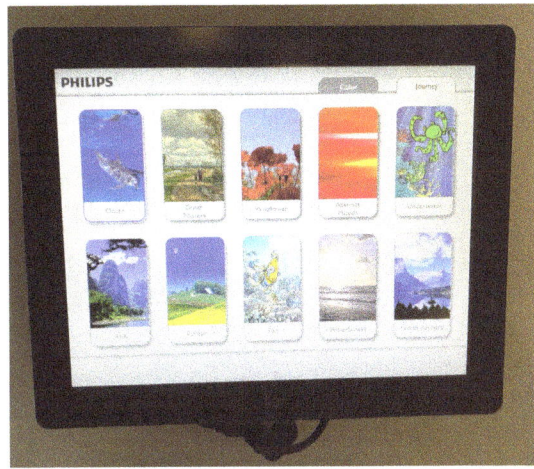

The MRI machine uses a combination of strong magnets, a radio transmitter, and a receiver. When the imaging sequences are performed, electric current is sent through a coiled wire. The switching of the currents causes the coils to expand, which makes the loud clicking or banging sounds we hear.

To me, I imagined the banging was just bubbles popping as they reached the surface of the aquarium.

CHAPTER 12

PROSTATE SIZES AND PIRADS LESIONS

From my study I new that a normal prostate measures about 3*3*5 cm and is about the size of a walnut. My measurements were 5.4 x 3.9 x 4.8 cm. The narrative from the MD Tech that reviewed the results stated "IMPRESSION: PIRADS 4 lesion in the left mid gland peripheral zone. No evidence of extracapsular extension, neurovascular bundle invasion, lymphadenopathy, seminal vesicle invasion, or osseous metastatic disease."

It went on to say, "Lesion 1: Within the left mid gland peripheral zone at the 3:00 position there is a low T2 signal lesion on series 5 image 17 measuring 0.4 x 0.3 cm with corresponding low ADC map signal on series 6 image 17. In craniocaudal dimension, this measures 0.4 cm series 3 image #9. This is a PIRADS 4 lesion. Other pelvic findings: Trabeculated bladder suggests chronic partial bladder outlet obstruction in the setting of BPH. Minimal diverticulosis of the colon is questioned on the left series 3 image 2 without diverticulitis."

At the time, I had no clue what all this meant. In hindsight, and now knowing more, the key takeaway items were that from the tech's viewpoint, there was a PIRADS 4 lesion in the left mid gland peripheral zone (that means cancer). However, there was no tumor growth beyond the prostate into the surrounding soft tissue, which was good!

He did use the word "chronic" in describing my bladder outlet obstruction. I should have asked for a refund for that part of the

MRI exam, as I could have told him that fact from staring at the bathroom walls every hour over the years.

Something told me, however, from the looks of that expensive machine that they don't do refunds!

What does PI-RADS mean?

PI-RADS 2 – Low (clinically significant cancer is unlikely to be present).

PI-RADS 3 – Intermediate (the presence of clinically significant cancer is equivocal).

PI-RADS 4 – High (clinically significant cancer is likely to be present).

PI-RADS 5 – Very high (clinically significant cancer is highly likely to be present).

Mine was a PIRADS 4 lesion and that was a number I did not like to hear.

CHAPTER 13

DEBRIEF AND THE CANCER CONVERSATION

When I returned to Dr. Scott's office for the debrief, the upshot of the conversation, with a doctor I really liked, was presented to me from a high level, meaning not a lot of technical medical language. He told me "Yes, you have cancer; however, it looks like it could be contained." He continued by saying, "We need to do another test to see where cancer specifically is and to help make decisions as to the next steps, including the treatment."

He said he wanted to schedule an ultrasound-MR fusion biopsy. All I heard was that he used that word biopsy, and once I heard that, the snake was all I could think of.

An MRI/ultrasound fusion-guided biopsy combines a specialized magnetic resonance imaging (MRI) scan with an ultrasound image to help urologists precisely target the area of the prostate that needs to be biopsied.

On April 4, 2018, I arrived for my visit with the snake.

This procedure was done in the main hospital, and the wife came with me. This visit was a little more formal than what my first doctor had presented me with, as I had a nice waiting room with no Viagra posters on the walls. After a short meeting with the very nice patient access specialist, they wheeled me back to a patient room and told me to strip down, which is what I was expecting. The nurse started an IV, then a young man came in. He looked to be about twenty-four, but I know he had to be older. He announced he would be my anesthesiologist for the day

DEBRIEF AND THE CANCER CONVERSATION

and was going to give me something to relax. *O cool*, I thought, *this will be easier if I am going to be given some drugs to relax.*

When he put the shot in the IV tube, it was the last thing I remembered. I woke up in recovery and felt pretty good, with no blood and gore like my other two trips to the snake, and my cheeks were not all slimily. So I headed home with the wife driving.

Looking back on this visit with the snake, I'm not sure but I don't think I was ever told I would be put under. That was not that big of a deal but would have relieved a lot of stress for me several days leading up to the procedure, so ask your doctor if you will be taking a nap during the procedure!

Waiting for the results of the Biopsy and knowing I had a PIRADS4 score my mind was giving me vibrant dreams of going through all kinds of doors in a big house and seeing different scenarios play out. I would have this same dream again in a few years but about a different person.

My results came back on April 6th, and I headed back to see the doctor.

As he talked to me, I was already apprehensive. After all, the PIRADS 4 lesion already told me that there was something there and I don't care who you are, your mind can talk to you in strange ways when you know you have cancer.

As he talked about the procedure results, I noted him saying twelve biopsy samples had been taken, and for one he used the word Carcinoma.

Dr. Scott explained to me that Carcinoma is a type of cancer that begins in cells that make up our skin, or it can also be the tissue lining organs; in my case, the prostate. Like other types of cancer, carcinomas are abnormal cells that divide without control, and they can spread to other parts of the body. Spreading is not a good thing to hear, as your mind will start to take you places where I would suggest a slap across the face and some positive self-talk is required.

I tried to focus on what the doctor was saying about sample number ten, where the report said "Prostate, left apex, needle core biopsy: prostatic adenocarcinoma, Gleason score 7 (3+4), grade group 2, involving 5% (1 mm) of one core." All the other eleven samples were benign. The report went on to say, "Doctor XXX (redacted) has reviewed slide 10A-L3 and concurs in the diagnosis of Adenocarcinoma."

The reality was I had no clue what all of this meant. I mean I was hanging on, understanding a little of the data. I knew that the word benign was good but had no clue about the word adenocarcinoma or what a Gleason score was. For that matter, I didn't know we were keeping score. All I knew was several folks had concurred that I had cancer!

What I now know is that adenocarcinoma (ad· e· no· car· ci· no· ma) is a type of cancer, with common types including breast, stomach, lung, colorectal, and, in my case, prostate.

Dr. Scott said we should discuss this in more detail and suggested that I go home for a few weeks and think about what I wanted to do. I was like, *Go home and think about it?* I'm like, *I'm good! Let's get rid of it today!* However, I did as he instructed and went home with the news.

On the drive home, the "O shit, I really have cancer in me" hit. My thoughts drifted to time to make a will; talk to my pastor; go bungee jumping. Heck with bungee jumping, let's go base jumping and fly a hang glider. Then at the next stoplight, I slapped myself and remembered I already do those things, and I remembered what my brother told me. "This too shall pass" and so I continued home to think about it.

CHAPTER 14

I DIDN'T KNOW WE WERE KEEPING SCORE

The Gleason score is just that, a score or grading range developed by Dr. Don Gleason who who was a pathologist at Minnesota University medical school. I learned that originally, there were five grades, from one to five. Grade one lesions were the most deafferented and grade five the least differentiated. Prostate cancers tend to be heterogeneous (diverse in character or content), with two or three grades within a prostate gland. When the pathologist grades what they are seeing, the ranges are from one to ten, with a score given for a primary and a secondary. This describes how the pathologist sees cancer when looking at biopsy specimens under a microscope; healthy tissue is a lower score, while abnormal tissue equals a higher score.

Two to six is ok, that is if you can call any cancer ok. It means the cancer is likely to grow very slowly. If the cancer is small, many years may pass before it becomes a problem. So, you may never need treatment.

Seven means the cancer is likely to grow and spread, hopefully at a modest pace. If the cancer is small, several years may pass before it becomes a problem. To prevent problems, however, treatment is needed.

Eight to ten means the cancer is likely to grow and spread fast if not already. If the cancer is small, a few years may pass before it becomes a problem. Generally, treatment is needed right away.

What I know now, and you should pay attention to if you hear these numbers, is that my Gleason score of seven was a 3+4. Understand that this is different from 4+3, I know it's new math but, those are two different ways to get to seven. Neither is good, but 3+4 is better than 4+3. Even now, three years later and as I am trying to renew my life insurance (try to get life insurance at sixty-two after having cancer and being a pilot too), the insurance underwriters are telling me with a 3+4 the cancer is less severe and they should be able to help me (it's going to be expensive), but not if it was a 4+3.

Once you have this talk with your doctor, and have the scores and biopsy results, the questions you are supposed to answer and the calculations you need to make go as follow. OK, I have a seven (either 3+4 or a 4+3) so is the cancer small? How do you measure small when something is growing inside you? Growing indicates getting larger. What kind of day was the pathologist having when they did my review? Did they have a hangover, or miscount something while looking in that microscope? Did they sneeze and say whoops and just write down a number? How the hell am I supposed to decide on having or not having a major surgery based on a lot of "ifs"? And what exactly is the definition of "slow-growing"? Do we put a window in our abdomen so we can look each day and calculate our odds of it spreading to other parts of our bodies where it can't be stopped? Is there a trigger or warning a few days before it spreads as a last warning?

A few days later, I was visiting my parents and decided not to tell them what was up. While there, I talked with my brother's wife about my possible prostate cancer, she is a very talented and experienced nurse with all kinds of credentials. Her response was, "Heck, just cut it out." It sounded reasonable to me, easy breezy right? At least it sounded that way.

What I figured was cutting it out sounded better than a visit to the Snake each month?

CHAPTER 15

OPTIONS AND CRITICAL DECISIONS

A few weeks later, I was rested, my head was in a better place, and I came back to see Dr. Scott. As we talked, he again described several options based on the MRI and biopsy results.

Waiting and monitoring

Radiation therapy

Chemotherapy

Removal of prostate via surgery

Dr. Scott did not try to lead me toward any answer or treatment, or any specific way of looking at things. I felt our talks had very low pressure but was a very fact-oriented conversation. I could feel he genuinely wanted the best for me. The options I liked came down to waiting and monitoring the growth or having it taken out. The waiting and monitoring sounded good to me, as I was always prone to procrastination. After all, I wasn't sick and why would anyone volunteer to get cut on and have parts of their inner guts removed if not needed?

Then again, I flashed back, realizing that I would most likely have to visit the snake more often for more samples. I remembered the words from the tech on the MRI report, saying there was no tumor growth beyond the prostate into the surrounding soft tissue. I knew that growth outside of the prostate was not going to end well, as I thought about Rob, my hang-gliding friend who had died earlier, so I ask what would happen if I did nothing. The answer was swift, direct, and with confidence. "Most likely five to seven years of the good life"; and, if it spreads during those five to seven years, I ask. "Hard to say; it could be quick or could linger."

After a minute or two of calculations in my head, I decided dying like my hang glider pilot friend, who found out too late, was just not an option for me. I did not want to go down at a young age with all kinds of tubes and chemicals being pumped into me while flying all over the world for exotic treatments as a last-ditch effort. So, I elected door number two, radical prostatectomy via the robot.

The pro for me for robotic surgery was that once the surgery is over, you generally know where you stand. You hope that your PSA is zero, which means chances are that you are cured. The downside is that one wrong move of the robot, and fun, future sex is over! With radiation, the downside is that once you have the radiation treatment, it could be months or as much as a year before you know whether you've been cured or not. So, for me, surgery came out on top, and we scheduled the robotic surgery for August 21, 2019.

I believe you must have confidence in your doctor. I asked Dr. Scott if he felt confident in doing the removal and how many of these surgeries he had done (hey, you must ask, right?). He was very modest and said he had done quite a few and to feel free to look him up. I was already confident, but look I did and impressive was an understatement. I was embarrassed I had even asked the man, but you need to, and then you need to go look.

So, I used my vast internet skills and looked him up a little deeper.

Early 1990s–While in his residency (his program was an early adopter of advanced urologic laparoscopy techniques), Dr. Scott laid the foundation to become one of the first urologists to perform these procedures on a large-scale platform outside of an academic center.

1995–Performs my states first laparoscopic kidney removal for kidney cancer.

1996–First in my state to perform a successful complex reconstruction of the urinary tract (pyeloplasty and ureteral re-implant) via laparoscopy.

2000–Completes my states first laparoscopic prostate removal without robotic assistance. Less than 1% of urologists have completed one successful prostate removal in this manner, let alone several hundred, as in the case of Dr. Scott.

2003–Conducts my states first prostate removal using a robotic surgery system.

2005– Develops the S.P.E.C.I.A.L™ (sequential pre-emptive exposure of cavernosal innervation with atraumatic ligation) surgical technique for preserving nerve function after prostate removal, which improves post-operative erectile function. Not only does this technique protect the essential nerve bundles, but also the surrounding neural structures and supporting tissues prone to injury from the slightest manipulation.

Present–Performs more than 250 various robotic surgeries and laparoscopic procedures every year, and continues to provide education to other physicians through a peer-reviewed journal, book chapter publications, hands-on teaching, and scientific presentations. He is also an accomplished musician and composer who has written a variety of songs (including a new one about the emotional impact of a cancer diagnosis).

My wife was correct; this man was badass!

CHAPTER 16

THE DAY OF CUTTING APPREHENSIVE BUT CONFIDENT

August 19th was a Monday and the day of surgery. The morning of the surgery, the doctor came in while I was being prepped and asked how I was feeling. I told him I was apprehensive but very confident. He thanked me for my confidence in him, and I was rolled into a big room.

I love technology, so the da Vinci surgical robot was cool-looking to me with all its arms. I could see the command station or terminal positioned slightly away from the operating table. This is where my doctor would be seated, most likely listening to some cool jazz all while driving the beast.

During all our conversations, I knew about the robot but wasn't told exactly what would happen during the actual procedure. I know now this surgery is a major deal. There is a series of videos of actual surgery you can watch on YouTube. Just Google prostate surgery and you'll find several. I have now watched them and would suggest you do too; just don't watch the first two because they are kind of gross.

I thought I had thought of everything and was ready until I was actually there for the surgery, and it was about to happen. There is a point where you have to self-talk to yourself, saying, "Ok, these folks are professionals; this doctor is sharp; in fact, he is the best of the best so what possibly could go wrong? They do a lot of these surgery things now; this is 2019 and medicine is solid science, right?"

The surgery began with all the folks in the room going through the necessary protocols. I remember laying on the table as the light conversation in the room turned very professional. The announcements by the surgical staff of, who I was and what was about to happen started. Then someone said "Ok, let's begin."

Trying to lighten the mood, I chuckled and spoke up, asking, "Are you using Propofol? Who invented that anyway?" There

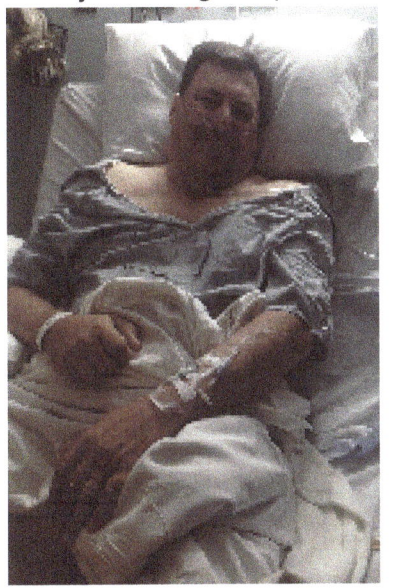

was silence but just as the lights in my head were starting to dim, the last thing I remember hearing was someone speaking up and jokingly saying, "Michael Jackson."

Five hours later I woke up, and everything was fuzzy, I was starting to figure out where I was as things came into focus. There were a couple of folks in the room that said, "Hi Mr. Whitney, welcome back, how do you feel?" My wife was there, and I remember saying out loud, "Well, I don't see velvet fabric or dirt so everything must have gone okay!" The nurses were laughing at that statement.

The care I received from these fine nurses was excellent and I was told the surgery went well. I felt beat up and groggy, but they said that was normal after having seven holes cut in me and my belly blown up seven to ten times normal size so a robot can shine lights, poke, prod, and cut on me.

In the United States, about 90,000 radical prostatectomies are performed each year and an estimated 70,000 are performed, like mine, robotically. [3]

Before surgery, I was not aware of the amount of trauma that was going to happen to my body, which was most likely a good thing. I knew that Dr. Scott is an advocate and is known for reduced invasiveness and faster healing. Laying there in the recovery room, I thought a lot about having my belly expanded, stripped away from my guts to make room, and expose so the robot could get to it. The reality was, I felt pretty good and was not hurting!

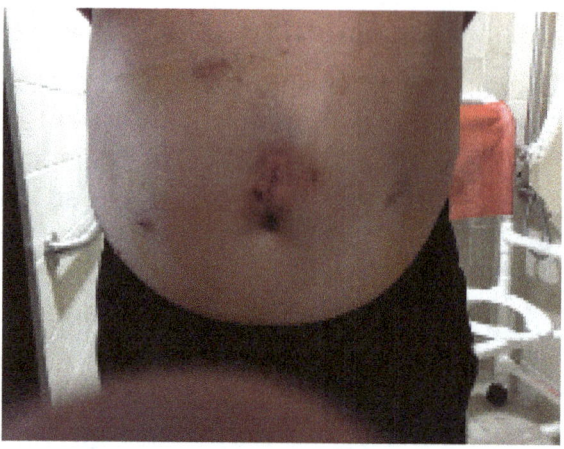

Dr. Scott stopped in later in the evening to chat with me. He said the surgery had gone well and the nerves were mostly saved. Without saying it, his words indicated I should be good for sex, which was, I assure you, not something on my immediate mind but was comforting to know. He said I could go home the next day if I felt up to it.

All during the night, the nurses gave me meds every few hours. I didn't question it as I was in and out of sleeping hard, most likely due to the pain meds. I overheard the nurses as they were changing shifts talking about how my blood pressure was so low and what should they do about it. Then I remembered in a couple of my awake moments when the meds came, I remembered they were giving me blood pressure medicine repeatedly along with the pain meds, and I should only have it once a day. Once I brought this up to the nurses, my BP returned to normal. So, pay attention and audit what you are being given while in the hospital.

I went home the next day, wheeled out in a chair and letting my wife drive home, which can be scarier than surgery. Recovery was not too bad; in fact, it was great, and Dr. Scott's reputation for non-invasive cuts and fast recoveries was intact. I had a large catheter inserted in my penis, and a bag strapped to my leg. It was uncomfortable but, overall, I felt pretty good. I had never had a catheter before and wanted to have a look at it but could not bend over far enough to see what it looked like or how it was hooked to me. I ended up using my phone to take photos so I could see what that was all about, which I don't suggest doing.

Three to four days after my surgery and being a business owner who was in the middle of moving my shop to a new location with a lot of construction under way I slid myself out of the easy chair and went to work. It was against the wife's wishes, but I said I was fine. I was slow and did not stay long each day, but I did it. I told myself I got this; having my prostate removed was not so hard at all.

After a few more days, a review with a new PSA test showed my PSA number was <0.1 ng/mL, so it appeared I had made the right decisions and got the cancer before it had spread. I was feeling cocky! This recovery, I thought, was going to be easy breezy.

CHAPTER 17

THE THING MEN FEAR THE MOST

During my recovery I remember having the catheter removed the most. A couple of weeks after surgery I called and told the nurse, "I want this thing out of me!" She said, "Sure thing. It's been long enough, come on in." My wife drove me to the doctor's, and little did I know she had been informed by one of my associates of how this would go. I knew the nurse well after all my visits because her husband was into hobbies, and they had visited my hobby shop before. I did not give much thought as to the procedure or how taking this rubber hose, which looked to be substantial, out of my penis was going to happen. I mean surgery was easy, the drugs were good, and I was recovering well, but this thing was a nuisance and had to go!

"Pants off, lay on the table," she said. By this point, stripping in front of doctors, even cute women were a non-issue for me. She was very conversational, chatting about her husband's hobby adventures. What I did not notice was she was wrapping her right hand around that rubber hose several times near the head of my penis, all while looking at her left hand that had moved to my groin to hold my penis. All I remember was her bending over and saying, "Let's look and see what we have here," and then she yanked it out without any warning! It felt like someone had reached in my penis up to my neck and pulled my head out the hole! I swear I saw stars while her arm stretched what looked like five feet with the elastic tube. There was so much hose up inside me, then pop and it was out. She quickly grabbed the strategically placed towels, as urine flowed everywhere.

THE THING MEN FEAR THE MOST

I would propose that catheters rank close to the top of the list of things all men fear. And since I have just emerged from having an XL size one pulled out of me, I'm here to tell you that those fears are valid. It's a nightmare. It's everything horrible you expect, and somehow worse.

I learned later that the tubing inside you is a little over nine inches long and can stretch a long way! Thank God it was quick, and that no one had told me what was going to happen.

After I regained some composure, I went to the potty with one of those female menstrual pads the nurse handed me with a smile. I was leaking profusely, and the aftermath was not comfy! After stopping by the front desk to schedule my next visit, and having somewhat composed myself, I came back to her station and gave her a big hug. I said, "I hate you but thank you so much for not telling me anything beforehand!" She looked at me with a big grin on her face. I limped down the hall out into the waiting room, my driver (wife) smiled and said, "How was it?" I later learned she knew what was going to happen and said nothing.

Have I mentioned I have a great wife?

CHAPTER 18

TIME FOR A BEER BUT WTF IS THIS?

That afternoon after the appointment, I was happy to be done. I plopped down in my easy chair and opened a beer. Life was about to be better. After a bit, I went to stand up and leaked what felt like the entire beer out into my pants. WTF! Dr. Scott had said I might have to wear a small pad, but I needed a bucket! I was leaking like crazy and had to rush in some Depend© guards for men. Tip: only get that brand. Do not buy the generic Kroger© brand, as they did not work at all (no absorption). After finding this out in the middle of the night, the wife made an emergency trip to find the good ones, or I was going to sleep on the toilet.

On September 24, 2019, about a month post-surgery, I was still leaking like crazy. I started to request more information on the Kegel exercises I was doing to help me recover. I was going through ten plus of those big pads a day. I was doing the Kegel exercises as per the directions, but the leaking was not getting better. This was worse than before surgery, at least then I got to pick the bathroom. Now I was in the bathroom, changing out soggy pads, ten times a day.

Five months later and six months after the surgery, on February 1, 2020, I sent an email to Dr. Scott that said, "I am seeing a little progress each week, slower than I anticipated but better all the time." The reality was I was hoping that being optimistic was going to help. I was prescribed some bladder control medicine to see if it would help.

However, on April 4, 2020, another note was sent: "Hi Dr. Scott. A few months ago, during my last visit, you prescribed some

TIME FOR A BEER BUT WTF IS THIS?

medicine that you said 'might' help with bladder control. I used it for the month until it ran out and 'think' it helped. It's been eight months since the surgery, and I am still having issues. I am good when sitting but if I'm standing or trying to walk to get back in shape, it is hard to control the bladder and I am always leaking. I am at seven plus pads a day (still the big ones), which is better than ten but this is very frustrating, and I hate going through life with wet pants. I am thinking about moving my desk into the bathroom ;-). Should I try those pills again? Will more exercise help this get better?"

That same day, I got a reply from a nurse that said, "Keep doing the Kegels. We can refer you to a physical therapist to help get you on track if you would like. I will have Andy send in a new Rx for the meds."

Looking back, if I knew before surgery what I would be experiencing now, eight months after the surgery, I am pretty sure I would have rolled the dice and taken the five to seven years. Hey, after all that, 3+4 was better than a 4+3, right?

CHAPTER 19

BLADDER CONTROL AND KEGELS

Kegel exercises are used to strengthen the muscles responsible for bladder control. These pelvic floor muscles are the same muscles you use to prevent urination or to keep from passing gas at an inappropriate moment. When you squeeze your anal sphincter, you are also squeezing your urinary control muscle.

How do you learn Kegel exercises?

These muscles should be tightened without tightening the abdominal, thigh, or buttock muscles at the same time. If you are not sure which muscles to tighten, the next time you urinate, try stopping the stream. Another helpful hint is to imagine that your doctor is performing a prostate exam; (I know that is not fun) envision you are squeezing the doctor's finger (anal sphincter) but not the buttock muscles. For those patients who still have trouble identifying the correct muscles, I am told your doctor can arrange computerized bio-feedback training under the direct supervision of a therapist.

How often should you perform these exercises?

The instructions I was given said, to do the exercise, tighten the pelvic floor for a slow count to five and then relax. Perform one set of ten reps three times per day (thirty total per day). With this intensity, any more often might over-fatigue these muscles and temporarily worsen your bladder control. After two to three

BLADDER CONTROL AND KEGELS

weeks of "training," the next step is to consciously contract these muscles when you are about to sneeze, cough, stand, or whatever causes your "stress incontinence" (actions that cause you to lose bladder control). As these actions become automatic, you will continue to see improvement in your symptoms.

When should you start?

Although some urologists recommend Kegel exercises immediately (even with the urinary catheter in place), I knew that Dr. Scott performs a very complex reconstruction of the pelvic floor to help ensure recovery of urinary function. To avoid disruption of this reconstruction, Dr. Scott usually recommends starting these exercises approximately four to six weeks following surgery. In some cases, quick recovery of urinary function eliminates the need for Kegel exercises.

CHAPTER 20

GRADUATIONS AND A TRIP TO CELEBRATE

December 2020, while in the middle of COVID and with me peeing in my pants every second of the day, my daughter Sierra graduated from college, early, and she was on the president's list too. She and I have the same birthday 11/07, only separated by time. We are both textbook Scorpios with strong passions and personalities to match. She is so smart and due to COVID, I was disappointed she did not even get to walk to receive her diploma, robbed after so much work.

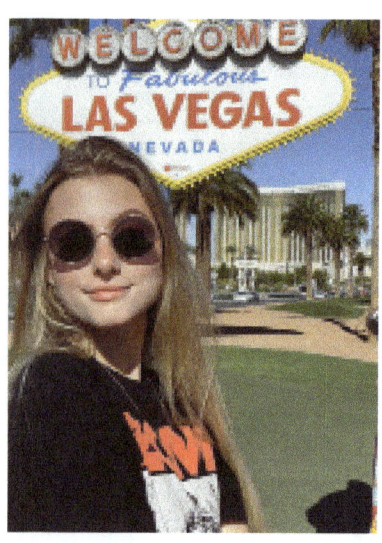

I posted a short note on social media the day her graduation was official and just before we headed to Las Vegas for the celebration of graduation and her turning twenty-one:

"There was once a little girl named Sierra. As much as her daddy fought it, she grew up into a strong woman, conquering the world with confidence and strength. Her daddy was a proud papa!

"Last night, her daddy was once again extremely proud as it was announced that she had completed her studies at the prestigious Kennesaw State University.

"Not just any completion, mind you, but with majors in integrated studies and criminal justice.

"Sierra graduated in style and in an elite group of only a very few, with great distinction, Magna Cum Laude!

"Sierra, we share a special day together, twins if you will, only separated by time. I think often of the miracle God has given moms and dads with the ability to create a life, but it comes with great responsibility and fear. I once asked my mother if she ever stopped worrying about her kids as we got older. She replied that 'she prayed a lot' and as for my life, I think she has a direct hotline.

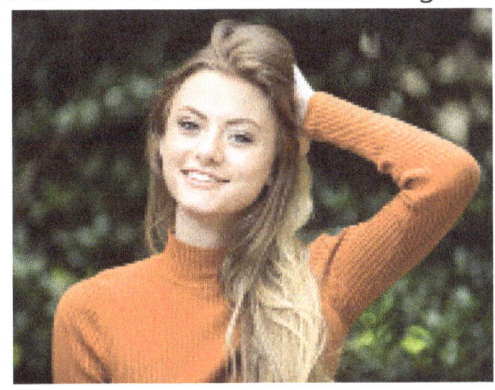

"A parent's responsibility continues as we do our best to set examples and teach our creation how to grow, explore, and live life in the largest way. As I look at photos of you growing up, our trips and experiences together, and as I live vicariously with your adventures traveling the world, I know just how blessed we both are.

"We are Scorpios. You are tough, and you are, as I am told I am also, intense, stubborn, and analytical but with tenacity, will-power, passion, and great faith. I always watch you from afar. You are smart with a strong, independent soul; kind, you are, and respectful to others, which will drive your success. Never lose these traits. Focus on them, live by them, and spread it around as the world needs more of it.

"I remember your first tooth, your first steps, your first bike ride, your first airplane ride, and the post-it notes you left on my computer as a little girl (still there).

"I am so very proud of you, Hot Rod. Congratulations on this, another epic achievement!

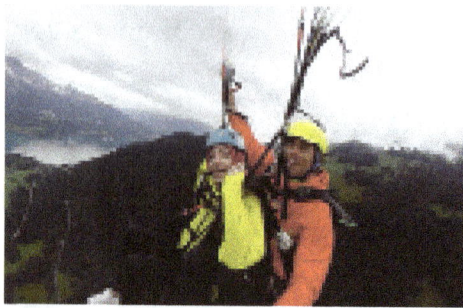

You now have time to focus and continue to discover your passion.

"Everyone, watch out; this one will change the world!

CHAPTER 21

MORE CANCER, MY BROTHER DIES

March 1, 2021: In the wee hours of the morning, I received a call from my niece in Charlotte. I had already felt it in my soul as I answered the phone with my hand shaking, before she coud say anything I said, "I know". My younger brother Scott had died of very aggressive lung cancer that spread to his spine and brain.

Eight months earlier, when he first called me with the news, I played the cool older brother and told him to be positive and

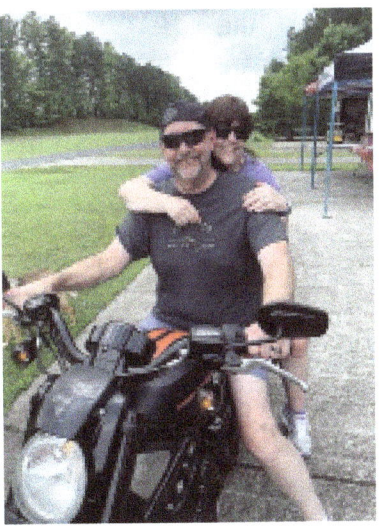

that based on my journey the medicine and surgeons were magic, and that it would be ok. What I did not know was that he was holding back the real news of it being terminal.

Scott and I were fortunate to be able to spend a lot of time together in the eight months from his diagnosis to the last night he went to sleep. He was always laughing and never complained as his condition worsened and as family boosted his sprits with hot dog-paloozas in his neighborhood and campfires at my hanger. Scott and I were able to ride motorcycles and drive my wife's Corvette like wild men in the mountains.

Scott spent many long weekends at my home where he was able to fly in my and my neighbors' experimental airplanes, doing aerobatics like professional air show performers. Each time he was asked if he wanted more "acro," he would reply, "Hell I'm dying anyway. Give me all you got!"

We were able to travel to remote mountain tops, sit all alone, and breathe the clean air at over 5000 ft. We reflected on our childhoods, told stories about our other two brothers, and his wishes for me to look after his children.

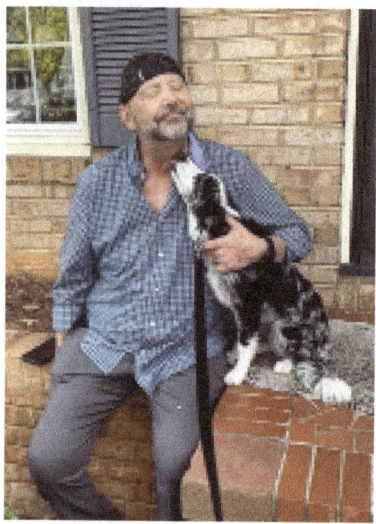

During these eight months, he took several trips with his wife and family to Hilton Head, the Florida Keys, and Cancun. His wife Tammy is a very talented nurse with a skill set to prove it BSN, RN, VABC, and CRNI to match. She was able to care for him at home where he wanted to be and where she administered his many medications. Scott was wearing fentanyl patches and taking a large group of other medicines to diminish the ever-growing pain, but he was always smiling and getting every bit of fun he could fit in each day. He even made fun of the fentanyl patches and told me "hey, when these things start to wear out just hit it with the hair dryer and you will get a bonus bump."

Scotts constant positive attitude made me stronger with my own battles and thankful for how early mine had been detected. His strength was powerful and empowering, he faced what he knew was coming and never complained, how could anyone be so strong?

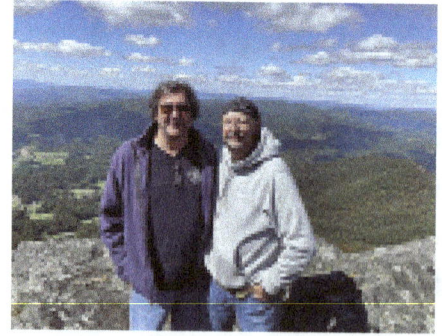

MORE CANCER, MY BROTHER DIES

His cancer was found late after having a persistent headache and getting some scans to see what was up, it took him way too quickly. I was blessed to speak his eulogy and tell the story of us as kids and to share a very vibrant dream I had had about a large house in heaven with unlimited doors to open and explore. It was standing room only because so many came to pay their respects.

Scott left a wife, two daughters, and a special video for his first granddaughter, born only a month after he entered heaven.

Until we meet again my brother, #belikescott

Cancer sucks!

CHAPTER 22

BABY DIAPERS AND CARRYING A LOAD

Two plus years have now passed since I was cut on, and I am still leaking like crazy. I am still up more than three times a night, and I can barely get a small erection, even using all the drugs which have nasty side effects.

Even after working hard with what felt like millions of Kegels (yes, I was doing them correctly), my only remaining sphincter just did not heal properly. I am leaking, a lot, and having to change the heavy-duty pads six to ten times a day, depending on my liquid intake, and I do try to limit what I drink, which is not a good thing to do. If you have ever seen a baby in diapers and he is carrying a load, that is what I feal like 24-7.

Those pads fill up, get heavy, and leak, getting you all wet just like those babies! My quality of life at this point was gone. I found I was staging those dam pads everywhere, in all the cars, coat pockets, in and around my desk, in a cabinet at my shop's bathroom, etc. Plus, this whole ordeal is just plain embarrassing, as these pads leak even when used properly (I have lots of experience now).

I tried everything, tight underwear and pants, and still, I leaked, and my pants got wet. I even quit drinking (drank nothing) for three days once to see what would happen. (Don't do that). I'm busy at work each day and found I was running to use a hairdryer or heat gun to dry out my pants and undies so I can keep a small semblance of a normal schedule, and God forbid if I try to go on a small hike or ride my motorcycle on a trip or fly our airplane. I would even keep a dry set of underwear and pants in the car or trusty backpack, as sometimes I would be so wet, I would have to go in the bathroom, strip, throw away the old, and change into the new.

Life was sucking, big time, and I wished this on no one!

CHAPTER 23

GETTING THE GUN OUT, I SIMPLY CANNOT GO ON LIKE THIS

On March 19, 2021, I was more and more depressed and so I went to see Dr. Scott again. I told him I simply couldn't go on like this. I said, "I have a balanced perspective, a good sense of humor, a great support system, and have done the hard work with persistence. What else is there or should I just get out the gun?"

I could tell by his face he was truly shocked. He said, "This is a very, very rare occurrence, one in thousands!" I had already researched some fixes, including more surgery, and asked about inserting a urethral sling. He said after about eighteen months, all the healing that was done was done and it would most likely not get better. He suggested I see a colleague of his that specializes in options for where I was currently in recovery.

Only about 6% of men who have their prostate removed have long-lasting incontinence. [4]

I learned that in healthy men operated on by an experienced surgeon (I had the best), about 80% should be wearing no pads—or, at most, a security pad to catch the occasional drop three months after surgery. At twelve months, 95% to 98% should be continent (no leaks). [5]

I learned reading various online forums that men have not one, not two, but three separate anatomical parts to control urine. There is a sphincter in the bladder neck, one in the prostate itself, and then there's the external sphincter below the prostate.

Radical prostatectomy knocks out two of these, leaving only the external sphincter to do the work of three, which is a hard job.

My mind was in bad shape and while the gun statement was a joke, for now, my hope was that with this referral to a trusted colleague of Dr. Scott, life could improve.

CHAPTER 24

TEN PADS A DAY & MEETING DR. AVALON

On March 23, 2021, I went to see Dr. Avalon; she was in the same medical group as Dr. Scott and highly respected. Yes, I looked her up online as well: medical school at UNC-Chapel Hill with residency at Yale-New Haven Hospital and fellowship at Vanderbilt. This woman was sharp! After some chatting about what was happening, she asks me to drop my pants, grabbed my balls, and said, "Cough." I said, "You really don't want me to do that," and she said, "Go for it." I said, "You really don't want me to" . . . and I peed all over her hand. I said, "I told you so!"

After the exam, her review paperwork said, "Mr. Whitney is a 61 y.o. male who is here for follow-up of stress urinary incontinence following retropubic prostatectomy for G 3+4= 7 pT2N0 disease with a negligible PSA (<0.1).

"Mr. Whitney states that following surgery he did experience some urinary incontinence. He states it got better and he was down to 5-6 pads per day. On a bad day he wears 10 pads per day—he reports he is having bad days more often than not. He is very active. He reports the pads are damp with occasionally soaked pads. Denies urinary frequency or urgency. He reports nocturia x's 3. Denies any dysuria or hematuria. Denies any issues with constipation."

During this visit, and as I had been doing my homework on the forums, I ask about having a urethral sling put in. She said it will not help me at my stage. I also ask about a fancy Emsella machine, which she said it is not covered by insurance, is expensive, doesn't/won't work, and to save my money. She said my best hope is for what was called an Artificial Urinary Sphincter or AUS.

So I went home to study, but having a mechanical implant really scared me.

CHAPTER 25

MOTORCYCLE TOURING AND PEEING ON BUSHES

In July of 2021, after a tremendous amount of planning, including mapping out stops and bathrooms, I took another motorcycle trip, this time with my wife as a passenger. We trailered the bike to Boulder, Colorado, put the truck and trailer in storage, and spent the next twenty days on the bike exploring the beautiful state.

This was tough for me, as by now I was in bad bladder shape, using a lot of pads every day. I had two packs of fifty-two pads each when we left Boulder, and my only savior was that you are not drinking much while driving several hundred miles a day on a motorcycle as you are driving and at awe of the sights.

We had luggage packed in both side and top compartments as well as strapped to the top of the luggage rack of our BMW K1600 touring bike. During the first day of the trip, we rode a loop-up canyon drive to Nederland, then to Winter Park, Granby and the Grand Lake area. We then entered Rocky Mountain National Park and rode to the 11,827 ft. top of Trail Ridge Road at Estes Park. It was an Epic day.

The next day, we left Boulder for the top of 14,260 ft. Mount Evans where there was still ice and snow. The Mount Evans Scenic Byway (Colorado Highways 103/5) is the highest, paved passenger route in North America—including Alaska, Hawaii, and California. It ends at 14,130 feet above sea level, or twenty feet higher than the much more famous and popular Pikes Peak Highway.

Leaving Boulder for the next nineteen days, we stopped in beautiful Fair Play and Buena Vista, then over the continental divide, 11,312 ft. Monarch pass and down to Crested Butte. It sucked but all of these were also planned bathroom stops. From there on to Ouray, the Switzerland of the Rockies, where we stayed a few days to enjoy the hot springs.

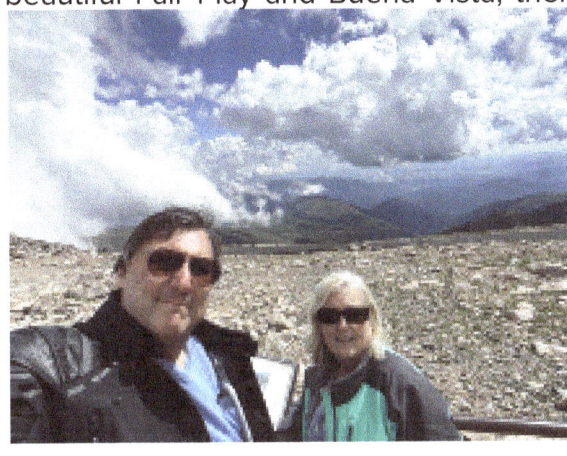

While there and at the suggestion of a good friend and neighbor (thanks Doug), we took a day and rented a 4WD and rode the Alpine Loop up over the continental divide and the 12,000 ft. Engineer and Cottonwood pass.

Colorado's Alpine Loop is a historic dirt road (kind of) and has a narrow window in which it's snow-free (June to September). But it's worth the wait—the sixty-five-mile scenic drive travels through a surreal landscape of treeless tundra and mountains that look like they are sprayed with red and yellow paint. You can access it from Ouray, Lake City, and Silverton. It's important to note that the entire route is four-wheel-drive terrain, so if you're piloting the family sedan, you may want to consider switching to a higher-clearance vehicle before attempting this magnificent route.

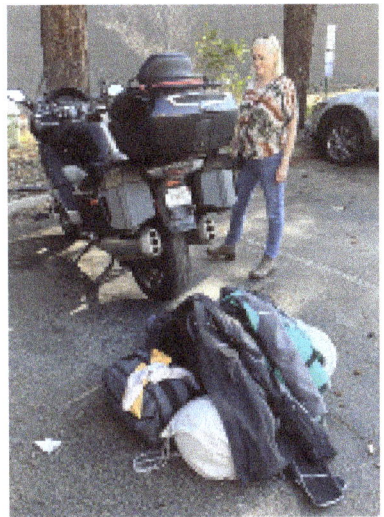

After the Alpine Loop, it was back on the bike, riding to Silverton, down to Durango, and spending a few days in beautiful Telluride before heading to Aspen for a few days where we met up with my son Eli and his girlfriend Ruth. From Aspen, we rode back over the continental divide in wet and freezing road conditions over 12,095 ft. Independence Pass to Leadville, passing by Breckenridge, and back to Boulder, then to Denver where we stayed one more night before loading up and starting the long drive home.

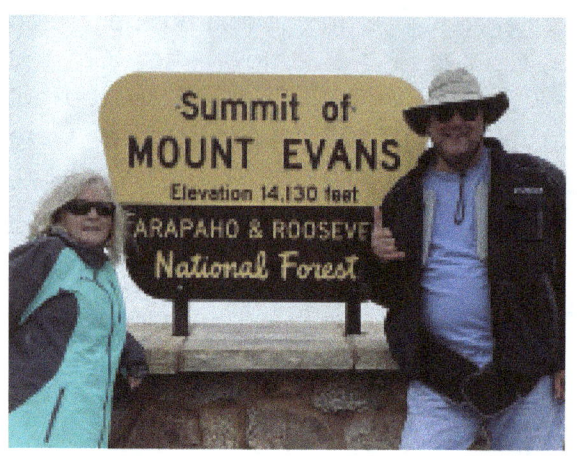

This trip was so much fun for us but tough on me, as there are not too many bushes to hide behind or pee on at 14,000 ft.

CHAPTER 26

LOSING A CHILD AND MAKING DECISIONS

I was still trying to decide if I should go forward with the AUS surgery. Months had passed since I last talked to Dr. Avalon and some days I just thought it would be so nice to just go to sleep and not have to deal with the embarrassment of being wet any longer. It was September 15th, 2021: and this morning, I lost my third child and my best friend. I was devastated. Katana Jean Whitney was 112 years young she was everyone's best friend.

I tell my kids to live large, and Katana did just that. Her story is that she was found in a box next to a major highway, with a bunch of brothers and sisters, as a very young puppy. Some ass had just put them out and left them to die. She was the runt, and my daughter Sierra fell immediately in love and named her Katana, telling me she needed an airplane name.

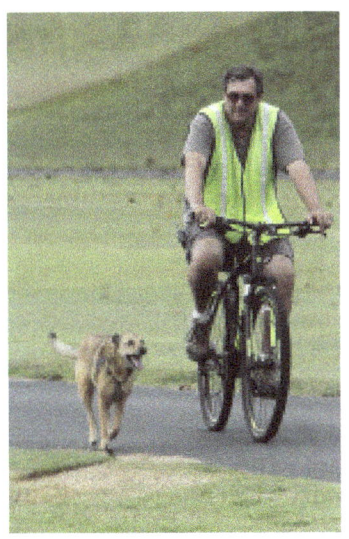

Katana was very social and loved to meet new people. She came to work with me at the shop every day, helped out in the shipping department, and was in love with the crinkle and texture of the big piles of brown paper, even putting some in her bed at times.

When my son and daughter were little, they would build forts out of the shipping boxes in the back of the shop and Katana was always in on the action. In her younger days, she was so strong and very fast. One time I clocked her at over thirty mph, and she would pull the kids on their roller blades around the runway at our home.

When little kids would come into the shop, she would greet them, and if she sensed they were scared of her, she would lay down and roll over, showing her belly to indicate she was chill. And chill she was, always smiling and just loving life and everyone at the shop and our neighbors at our airport home community called Stoney Point.

Many moms and dads have thanked me, telling me that their children were afraid of dogs but once they met Katana, the kids insisted to visit her at the shop often. Once she met you, she would never forget and would always greet you with a big smile.

Katana was a sponsor of the Forsyth Humane Society and often donated small drones and other hobby products to their auctions to help raise funds for other rescues. She loved to play in the snow, eat cheese fries and Chick-fil-A at the drive thru where everyone knew her. She loved to travel and ride in the car, and especially be on our camping trips to the mountains and lakes.

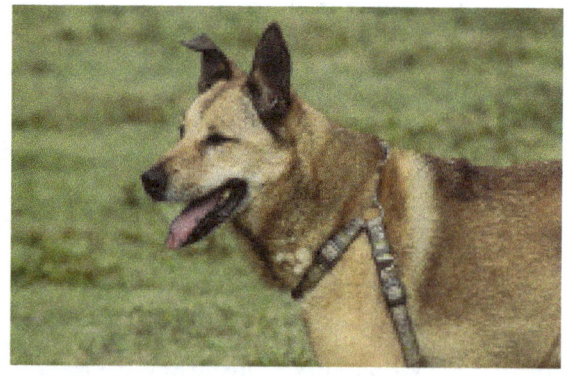

Katana was very old, her legs were failing, and she was just tired. On what only I knew was her last night, I spent time sleeping with her and brushing her with her favorite comb. She was very relaxed. All week she was having troubles and was letting me know it was time. I had been giving her medicine to help her pain. This morning, she slept late and when she got up, I lifter her into the truck and we went to Chick-fil-A for her favorite breakfast. We sat in the garage together, looking out at the light rain and I gave her an extra dose of medicine to relax. I had arranged for the very, very kind Dr. Erin Doiron at Alpharetta Animal Vet Hospital to come to the house. Katana knew and was ready; there was no pain. I held her in my lap, sitting in a chair talking to her and brushing her as we looked out over the runway, her favorite place.

I miss you so much every day, Katana. I know we will meet again and know your legs are strong again; you can hear again and see clearly; your mind is sharp, and you are running faster and faster with that big smile.

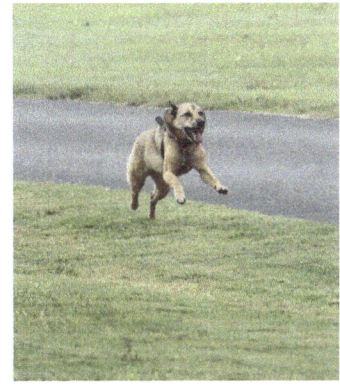

Our animals are much like we are, sometimes they are better than our kids (joking). They are always happy to see us and sometimes they get sick, and the medicine just does not work. Sometimes they, like us, are sad, sometimes they just get old and like us shut down or shut out the outside world. Like Katana, I was feeling old and down, the medicines and surgery had not worked, and I was feeling down, way down.

CHAPTER 27

NO OTHER OPTIONS SO SUCK IT UP!

For some reason, I kept hoping things would get better; it was almost a year after my first meeting with Dr. Avalon and three years after my prostate removal. My life was beyond unbearable. I was aware enough to know I was depressed and was having to talk to myself all the time to keep my mind in the proper attitude, mostly in the bathroom, so on January 21, 2022, I sucked it up and sent the following message to Dr. Avalon:

"Hi, Dr. Avalon, I hope you had a great Christmas and New Year with your family! We met at the direction of Dr. Scott last March, and after I peed on you, we had a conversation about the artificial urinary sphincter AUS.

"After doing a lot of study on the various message boards including,

https://www.ncbi.nlm.nih.gov

https://csn.cancer.org/discussion

https://forum.nafc.org,

I am now most likely your worst nightmare ;-)

"I have posted my story on two of these boards and have asked very pointed questions. The answers from those who have responded are positive but scary, nonetheless.

"With my study, if you will indulge me, I have a few questions.

1. How many AUS are installed in the USA each year?
2. To me, it looks invasive. I am reading it last only five or so years, rubs you raw, and there is a large chance of infection. Am I reading into this correctly?

3. The failure rate appears to be 30+%. With your experiences, would you agree with these #s?
4. Is the AMS 800 the device of choice? It looks like there are some new designs out of Switzerland, Europe, and even Argentina, and I am seeing some that are remotely controlled.
5. Will I have to have a catheter?
6. Recovery looks to be about six weeks before activation? What does activation entail? I am reading it can be painful.
7. How many of these surgeries have you performed over the last twelve to twenty-four months?
8. Am I reading too much into this, is it an easy-breezy surgery and I should not think twice about it?
9. What am I not asking that I should be asking?"

Her reply was quick, "Yes, you have been doing your homework. Please come see me so we can talk in detail."

On February 9, 2022, I headed to her office, again with questions in hand. We had a long, good conversion and I got to see the AUS (a sample) for the first time. It looked scary to think that this thing was going to be implanted in me. Dr. Avalon, like Dr. Scott, was not rushed, and there was no pushing to do a surgery, but I understood this was the only solution. I had to do some more thinking, so I went home.

A few days later, I sucked it up and with no other options, knowing full well that this would most likely be painful having a surgeon cut you from just above your asshole through your scrotum, with another cut in your belly to implant a mechanical pump called an AUS, I called to schedule the surgery.

March 17th at one pm was the day.

CHAPTER 28

CAMERAS UP YOUR PENIS

Before the surgery, Dr. Avalon required that she have a lookup inside my penis at my bladder to be sure there were no surprises when cutting me open. That sounded like loads of fun. NOT! But I had to suck it up. I asked, "How is this done?" She said, "The procedure is called cystoscopy and uses a long, thin, flexible, lighted tube called a cystoscope. I put a little camera at the end of a very thin catheter up your penis." I kind of tightened up and replied that sounds like fun I didn't want to have, and was there a door number two? "There's some discomfort, but you'll be fine." I knew full well that was a lie. When doctors say discomfort, I hear the 2004 horror movie *Saw* that my wife loves!

Doctors use terms that are related to you below the actual feeling to describe your upcoming predicament. "Discomfort" means pain. "Some pain" means really bad pain. "Light stinging" means a horrifying burning sensation and "pressure" means a weather balloon will be inflated inside of you.

After not sleeping due to knowing what was going to happen to me, I went into the office to have the camera put in me. The nice nurse took my blood pressure and announced, "It's a little high." I responded, "You think? You do know why I'm here, right?" She just laughed and had me strip and lay on a table. She stated, "I am going to give you a little anesthetic called lidocaine." I was hoping for a shot in the arm but instead, I heard, "You're going to feel a brief light sting" and then I get a needle pushed into the tip of my penis! Yea... read the paragraph above where I list a definition of "Light stinging".

CAMERAS UP YOUR PENIS

Dr. Avalon came in, all chipper-like and smiling, saying, "You ready?" She placed what felt like a cup over my penis, and I felt some suction. Then she said, "I need more water." It was then I understood that there was water being pushed up into my bladder as a tube was being run up in me, and she was looking into a small eyepiece connected to the camera. This was not fun; I was holding onto the sides of the metal table and then with my fingers intertwined on my chest, I was about to dislocate all ten fingers. The actual procedure only took about five minutes but in sheer horror, it felt like four hours!

Dr. Avalon announced, "Everything looks great. Your bladder looked a little small (I could have told her that and saved this trauma), but we are good to go with the AUS install."

CHAPTER 29

INSTALL DAY, I WOULD APPRECIATE WAKING UP

March 17th, one pm: not much sleep, knowing what was going to happen, and thinking about getting cut on again. I was wishing that we had done it earlier in the morning. Dr. Avalon came into the prep room where I was being taken care of to say hi and check in. As a joke, I asked her if she had been out drinking the night before. She smiled and rubbed her belly, as she knew that I knew she was eight months pregnant. She was upbeat and was laughing at my jokes, as I tried to reassure myself this was going to work out okay. She asked me how I was feeling, and I said my standard line for surgery, "Apprehensive but very confident!" The anesthesiologist said hi and ask me the usual questions like have I ever had a reaction that caused trouble. I assured him I had always woken up and that I would appreciate the same kind of service on this trip.

As I was wheeled into the surgery room, I noticed a lot of folks in the operating room. She had told me that when installing an AUS, the manufacturer rep must be present during the operation. These things are controlled pretty tightly; you just can't get one at the local department store. There are some very delicate measurements of your urethra to make sure the collar is the correct size and, apparently, the rep is the one to hand off the correct parts to the surgeon. My guess is there are also some liability concerns. I reminded her to please measure twice and cut once!

INSTALL DAY, I WOULD APPRECIATE WAKING UP

The operating room was different from the other one I had been in, as it appeared much larger. I saw Dr. Avalon checking some equipment, then the anesthesiologist put a mask on me and asked me to breathe deeply. I assumed this would put me out; however, it was just oxygen. Then as something was put in my IV, I heard someone say, "He is a good breather." I woke up three hours later now a cyborg with an implant in me.

I was very groggy during the initial recovery in the hospital. The nurse kept saying my heart rate needed to stabilize but I came through okay. I stayed in recovery an hour or so, until my wife came in and it was time to go. Yes, they can cut you from butt to balls, slice you in the belly, pull an implant between the two cuts, and send you home all in the same day. I least expected dinner for this $100,000 visit. ;-)

Getting off the recovery table was tough. I had been cut in a place where no man wants to be cut. I kind of slid off the table, not putting any weight on my ass, propping myself up with my elbows and waddled, very slowly with my balls in one hand, the few steps to the wheelchair, with a nurse on one side and my wife on the other. I think I said something to the effect of "no sex tonight!" The wife drove me home, and the next three days were pure hell. I was told recovery would be at least six weeks. Oh, how I looked forward to it.

CHAPTER 30

I'M ONE OF 5000 OUT OF THREE MILLION

The AUS is a cuff that is placed around the urethra. There is a pump placed in the wall of the scrotum, which is manually squeezed when you need to go. When you squeeze the pump, fluid is shifted from the cuff to a reservoir that is implanted behind the abdominal muscles below your belly. The movement of fluid allows the cuff to open, thus resulting in the opening of the urethra, allowing the flow of urine. The cuff spontaneously closes as fluid returns from the reservoir to the cuff. When the cuff is closed, the urethra is compressed again, and leakage is generally eliminated or reduced to a minimum.

The first artificial urinary sphincter to resemble the current model was developed by Dr. Brantley Scott in 1972. Called the AS 721, it consisted of a fluid reservoir, an inflation pump, a deflation pump, and an inflatable cuff with four unidirectional valves. [6]

The current AMS 800™ Artificial Urinary Sphincter was first released by Boston Scientific (formerly American Medical Systems) in 1988. Their product details state "is a completely concealed, implantable, fluid-filled, solid silicone elastomer device that treats male SUI resulting from intrinsic sphincter deficiency following prostate surgery. It mimics normal sphincter function by opening and closing the urethra at the control of the patient." [7]

Two hundred thousand patients have been treated with an AUS since 1988. So, my math says that 1988-2022 = thirty-four years, and that equals about 5,882 AUS installed a year. This sounds like a lot until you consider there are 90,000 radical prostatectomies done a year and, since 1988, that equals 3,060,000 performed so the AUS is installed in only 0.19% of patients. [8]

With this data, I am thinking I need to start a secret society complete with a covert handshake and all the other goodies a secret society brings. ;-)

CHAPTER 31

GREEN PEAS AND UNDERSTATEMENTS

My discharge notes after surgery by Dr. Avalon, MD 3/17/2022 stated the following:

No showering for forty-eight hours.

After forty-eight hours, you may shower. Do not scrub incision. You may pat dry incision

No soaking in tubs or swimming for four weeks.

No strenuous physical activity (gym) for four to six weeks.

Please continuously pull the pump down into the scrotum so that it scars in place in the scrotum and does not rise into the groin area. (Please do this at least three times per day.)

For pain/discomfort and swelling, you may apply an ice pack ten minutes on and ten minutes off.

Please take pain medications as prescribed.

Please take a stool softener while on pain medications to avoid constipation. Call if you experience fevers >101.5, nausea, vomiting, persistent pain, drainage from the surgical wound.

You will go home with a foley catheter in place; this should remain to gravity drain at all times.

Leg bag should only be worn while up and walking.

When sitting and resting in bed, the large drainage bag should be used.

GREEN PEAS AND UNDERSTATEMENTS

You may see blood in the urine with the catheter in place; this can be normal. You may experience bladder spasms, which is normal with the catheter in place

Please call if you notice no drainage from the catheter for >2 hours, and if you experience large clots passing through the catheter, preventing the catheter from draining. Your foley catheter may be removed at home on Monday if the urine is clear.

March 19th (Saturday): I was sleeping a lot but responded via email to a phone call from the previous day to see how I was doing after surgery.

"Yep, it hurts like hell, just can't get comfortable. Using ice packs on and off (green peas are your best friend). Eating the oxycodone and Tylenol. Urine is clear. Sucks having to lay on my back. The pump feels like it is in right place but is hard to tell. Managed to walk down the hall and back but for sure can't sit. Guess I must have patience?"

March 21, 9:02 am, Dr. Avalon replies:

"It can be pretty uncomfortable. Would you like to come in today for an exam to make sure everything is healing, OK? Happy to see you. The catheter can be removed today if not done already."

March 21, 9:37 am, I replied:

"Thanks, but Uncomfortable = understatement of year :-)

I had a reaction to the oxycodone and the Tylenol. Quit taking both Sat. morning, as I was itching a lot and it was making me feel bad. I am better this morning (no itching) but have a slight persistent headache (any suggestions?). Still in bed but can kind of walk, just not fun. The catheter I took out last night (that was fun too) no more blood in the urine. Feels like the cuff could be tight, as it takes a bit of time to pee but guess things are just swollen from the trauma and it will get better?

I am for sure not going to ride my motorcycle for a while :-)"

March 21, 9:57 am, a message from Dr. Avalon arrived:

"There should be a dimple in the pump that's in the scrotum. If not, then the system may be 'activated' and the cuff inflated, which we don't want. If you are not able to tell, pls come in so I can assess. There can certainly be some swelling after surgery, but we want to make sure that the cuff is not inflated. Caffeine and hydration are the best for headaches, assuming a run-of-the-mill headache."

My thinking was, that based on her emails Dr. Avalon: "Was concerned that the AUS had somehow been activated (it was not). When it is installed, all the fluid is held in the reservoir and the cuff is loose. You need to wait about six weeks for everything to heal up before you can do what is called the activation process, which enables the fluid to squeeze the cuff around the urethra to stop the leaking. Healing, in my mind, was slow, the healing from prostate removal was much faster and easier but the area where these cuts are made are a man's worst nightmare and healing takes time and a lot of patience."

On April 8th, I had a quick office visit with Dr. Avalon to check how the incisions were healing. Everything was looking good. I was hoping to get it activated that day but was told I had to wait. I was back at work but sitting on a nice, gel-filled pad and sitting way forward on it. Nothing could touch my scrotum area, and I mean nothing. Half days were the norm for a few weeks, which was hard for me being a shop owner but the recliner in the afternoons was paradise.

CHAPTER 32

ACTIVATION DAY, I'M NOW A CYBORG

I visited Dr. Avalon on May 3rd for the activation of the AUS. My studies had said this could be painful so I was ready when the doc said that it could be uncomfortable! Remember, being uncomfortable in doctor talk equals pain!

The turn-on of the implant involves squeezing a hard part of the pump just before the squeeze bulb in your scrotum. It is a very hard squeeze that must happen for at least several minutes to allow the fluid to release into the full system. Your scrotum is slippery on the inside and out, so the pump is hard to get a hold of, even when using two hands. I laid on the table, and Dr. Avalon did all the work. The squeezing was so hard, and it slipped out of her hands several times. Better gloves with some gripping pads were retrieved and that helped. After slipping several times, and with there being no bullets to bite on, I was about to dislocate my fingers squeezing them together. The internal part being squeezed on was so hard it was cutting into me, causing a little bleeding on the outside of my scrotum. It felt like I was having a hole poked in me. At one point, I told her to just get some pliers but then, success, the activation was done!

She had me try working it lying on the table and I could do this but would need some practice. I left her office with the understanding to call with any issues and if not, we would do a video call on May 17th.

As I left Dr. Avalon's office after the activation, I walked down the long hallway with the fancy hospital carpet and out into the parking deck. About halfway down the long line of parked cars, I clicked the key fob and opened the door of my 2008 Toyota Tundra. It was a stretch to get up and in, and even at 6 ft. 2inch., I still had to grab the handle just inside the door, which was up high on the left side of the driver's compartment. From there, I pulled myself up and stepped into the cab. It was a long high step and I paused as I sat down in the seat. I had lost count of how many times I had been poked and prodded. I had had so many things cut on and shoved up every orifice of my body, but for the first time in almost 1,000 days, and under the strain of pulling up to get in my truck, I was amazed I did not pee in my pants.

CHAPTER 33

WHAT I FOUND ON THE OTHER SIDE OF FEAR

It's been a tough few years for me. I got cancer and lost my prostate, my brother, and my dog. I feel that I am on the other side now and have found some freedom!

I just had a follow-up video conference with Dr. Avalon and will see her again in a few months. When I first decided to go forward with the AUS surgery, I asked her how I would feel a few months after surgery. She said I would either love her or hate her. During our call, she asked how I was doing. I reminded her of our conversation and told her we were now in a serious courtship and were about to be married.

I have learned how to squeeze the little bulb when my body tells me I need to pee. It's tricky to do. I still sit on the toilet for control but am practicing standing up and think I drain better. I use one hand, reach down, and can squeeze the bulb. It takes a couple of squeezes to release, and it happens quickly so when you squeeze, be ready or you will get a hand full ;-)

I am now wearing the very light guards. I don't even know they are there, and I am not really leaking at all, well, maybe a drip or two if under a lot of strain.

To be leak-free and to be able to do something simple like drink a nice cup of ice water is life-changing. I even did 180 miles with my wife, Eli, and Ruth on the motorcycles last week with no issues.

I pray that the AUS holds up just as the Boston Scientific data suggests it will. I am told it could be five to ten years before a replacement is needed. On the forums I have read, it could be more, or it could be less. One fellow said he had to go in after only one year for an adjustment so that is still in the back of my mind, and I pray it stays there. If all goes well, in ten years, I will be seventy-three and will decide then, if there are troubles, if I want to undergo another eight weeks of hell.

The last three years have made me think that I had let my family down, as I just couldn't do a lot of the things I could before. To avoid leaking, I have been mostly sitting for three years and am very out of shape and have gained weight. But to be honest, all of this has reminded me just how lucky I am. I am starting to walk again, each day but losing weight will take time.

The reality is that I know I am blessed to be alive but am still not convinced that I needed to go down the prostate removal path at all. I was the one that decided to remove it, based on all the information that was presented to me and how I understood it. There was no pressure to do the surgery. I also don't think there were any problems with or during the actual surgery, but for some reason I just did not heal properly, and the numbers say my issue is very rare.

The good part is I am seeing everyday life in a new way. A light has been turned on, and I am just thankful God has given me more time. Being a small business owner is tough, but I am not taking things so seriously any longer; in fact, I just promoted a general manager to run the shop's day-to-day operations and think I am going to start taking more time off. I have seen the other side and am no longer fearful or sweating the small stuff.

I am enjoying working with the local middle and high schools, I love teaching aviation and just taught my first summer camp, teaching aviation-based programs so kids and adults can explore and find their passions in life. Passion, you know, is that thing that you do in your free time, early in the morning and late at night: that thing you love to read about, write about, think about: that thing you do when there's no one to impress, nothing to prove, no money to be made, simply a passion to pursue. I teach my students that when you find it, that's your heart, your guide, and they should embrace it and run toward it full steam!

So many with my same cancer did not catch it early enough or have not had the opportunities and brilliant surgeons I have had, and somehow, with this writing and more, I plan to pay my good luck forward.

My cancer was a Gleason score 7 (3+4), grade group 2, involving only 5% (1 mm) of one core. In the big picture, and now, especially with the ability to look back, I think of it as just a spot.

Would I have been ok if I had not removed it and just waited and watched? Only God knows the answer to that question and one day, given the opportunity, I plan to ask Him.

What I do know is the decision to remove my prostate set off a chain reaction over three-plus years, and now I am cancer-free, but a cyborg with a secret handshake.

If I had waited and it had spread, I would be entering year four of a three-to-five-year life sentence, and, for me, that was not an acceptable outcome.

I have great faith, and it helped me over the past three years. So, if you are reading this and are having to make decisions as I have made, remember that if you ever come to the edge of all that you know, and are trying to decide if you should step off into the darkness of the unknown, don't hesitate. Go for it and don't bother to look down, because with your faith, one of two things will happen: there will be something solid to stand on, or you will be taught how to fly.

ABOUT THE AUTHOR

Cliff Whitney knows he is a blessed man. He lives on a private grass strip airport in Cumming, Georgia with Gail, his wife of 40+ years, a cat, lots of deer, wild rabbits, and a few coyotes. He has two grown children whose life planning, passions, and careers are allowing them to travel the world.

He has more than forty years of senior management experience in wholesale, retail, online, and manufacturing with a proven record of leadership and success. He is innovative and self-directed, with strong communication and interpersonal skills.

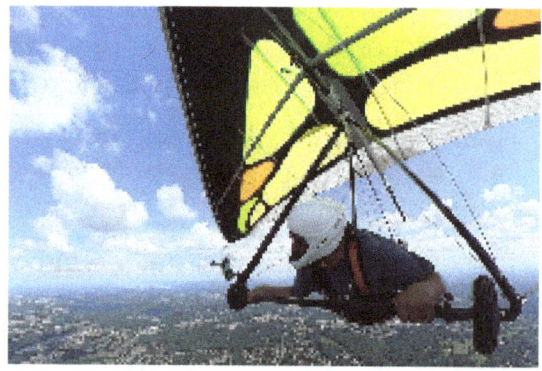

Starting as Whitney's Glider supply in 1978, his companies now specialize in remotely piloted vehicles and aerospace-related products. Previously, Cliff was the digital evangelist at Wolf Camera corporation. A twenty-four-year veteran of Wolf, he served in a number of sales, management, and senior management positions, as the company grew from five to over 700 stores across the United States of America. Cliff served as Wolfexpress.com's president, as well as Sr. VP of internet commerce and new technology development for the parent company.

When asked, "How do you measure success?" he says, "Aside from family, the easy answer is in the sales and profits that go to the bottom line and enable us to grow our business. The biggest success, however, is the chance I have to work with and grow talented groups of associates that will, in turn, grow themselves and change the world.

"The hobby and aviation industry, as well as photography and the now rapidly growing UAV/drone industry, are such emotional spaces; they touch lives and change the world at all stages. I feel very rewarded to know that we are and have been building products and enabling technology that can actually move society forward in a positive way, using science, technology, engineering, and mathematics. I am excited to be a part of this new frontier."

ENDNOTES

1 Chapter 2 paragraph 1

There is no known way to prevent prostate cancer. In the United States, data suggest it is the second leading cause of cancer death in men after lung cancer, which my brother Scott died of just a short time ago. Estimates are that over 34,000 men will die from this disease during 2022 in just the United States alone. So if you are diagnosed with prostate cancer late, and it has spread to other parts of your body, the five-year survival rate is 31%. For those of you that are not math-inclined, that is an almost 70% chance of dying.

Source https://www.cancer.net/cancer-types/prostate-cancer/statistics

2 Chapter 2 paragraph 6

Cancer, on the other hand, begins in the cells of where your cancer is. Around 400 BC, Hippocrates is said to have named masses of cancerous cells *karkinos*—Greek for "crab." Why a crab? If you feel a malignant tumor, you'll notice that it's hard as a rock. And so, it is thought that it reminded him of a crab's hard shell.

Source https://www.vocabulary.com/dictionary/cancer

3 Chapter 16 Paragraph 8

In the United States, about 90,000 radical prostatectomies are performed each year and an estimated 70,000 are performed, like mine, robotically.

Source https://www.onclive.com/view/robotic-assisted-laparoscopic-radical-prostatectomy-has-steep-learning-curve

4 Chapter 23 paragraph 4

Only about 6% of men who have their prostate removed have long-lasting incontinence.

Source https://my.clevelandclinic.org/health/treatments/8096-prostate-cancer-urinary-incontinence-after-surgery

5 Chapter 23 paragraph 5

I learned that in healthy men operated on by an experienced surgeon (I had the best), about 80% should be wearing no pads—or, at most, a security pad to catch the occasional drop three months after surgery. At twelve months, 95% to 98% should be continent (no leaks).

Source https://worldwidescience.org/topicpages/n/nerve-sparing+radical+prostatectomy.html

6 Chapter 30 paragraph 2

The first artificial urinary sphincter to resemble the current model was developed by Dr. Brantley Scott in 1972. Called the AS 721, it consisted of a fluid reservoir, an inflation pump, a deflation pump, and an inflatable cuff with four unidirectional valves.

Source https://emedicine.medscape.com/article/443737

7 Chapter 30 paragraph 3

The current AMS 800™ Artificial Urinary Sphincter was first released by Boston Scientific (formerly American Medical Systems) in 1988. Their product details state "is a completely concealed, implantable, fluid-filled, solid silicone elastomer device that treats male SUI resulting from intrinsic sphincter deficiency following prostate surgery. It mimics normal sphincter function by opening and closing the urethra at the control of the patient."

Source https://www.bostonscientific.com/en-US/products/artificial-urinary-sphincter/ams-800-artificial-urinary-sphincter.html

8 Chapter 30 paragraph 4

Two hundred thousand patients have been treated with an AUS since 1988. So, my math says that 1988-2022 = thirty-four years, and that equals about 5,882 AUS installed a year. This sounds like a lot until you consider there are 90,000 radical prostatectomies done a year and, since 1988, that equals 3,060,000 performed so the AUS is installed in only 0.19% of patients.

Source https://en.wikipedia.org/wiki/Artificial_urinary_sphincter

www.ingramcontent.com/pod-product-compliance
Lightning Source LLC
Chambersburg PA
CBHW050246220526
45465CB00002B/564